Praise for *All about the Burger*

"*All about the Burger*, is the Beast's love letter and tribute to America's favorite food, a cross between nostalgia, great history, and tidbits on how it became the star of American food. I truly enjoyed reading and connecting to my earliest memories of tasting a burger and a bite of the American dream."

—Ingrid Hoffmann, celebrity chef, author, and TV host

"We at Druther's anxiously await our copies of Sef's book in the mail. Sef was the *only* writer to reach out to our company regarding the history of Burger Queen, Huckleberry's and Druther's, as well as our company's relationship with the Dairy Queen brand. He also respected the unique story of the last Druther's Restaurant in the world, owned by our friend Steve McCarty, in Campbellsville, Kentucky. Sef's pursuit of the real story, along with the way he writes about the histories of these storied American restaurants and companies, truly conveys the respect and love he has for the subject."

—Bob Gatewood and Brian Easley, President & Vice President at Druther's

"With *All about the Burger*, the Beast has created—most fittingly—a thing of beauty. A book so meticulously researched and passionately written, it is the crowning achievement of one of our greatest food authorities. You will devour it instantly."

—Lee Schrager, Food Network's South Beach Wine & Food Festival, founder

"Read it for the sizzling burger history, stay for the tasty lore, the recipes and the juicy insider info that only the Burger Beast could

unwrap. Wherever you grew up in the US, you'll find the burger place of your childhood in delicious detail."

—Gretchen Schmidt, *edible* South Florida, editor

"For me, a mesmerizing page turner. I can't put this damn book down."

—George Motz, Hamburger America, author

"Some people look under the bun to see what's on the burger, Beast looks right through it, the toppings and the patties to determine where it lands on the overall historical arc of the sandwich, in all of its mouth-watering glory. I have been listening to his flavorful burger anecdotes for years and now they have been collected together and cleverly presented in one nicely bound book. Beast is the undisputed king of burger history...insert trademark here."

—Randy Fisher, CREaM, owner

"Burger Beast Sef Gonzalez leaves no bun unturned in this detailed look at the humble burger's rise to becoming America's iconic dish. I can think of no better chronicler for this meaty story than the man whose passion for burgers is boundless."

—Michael Mayo, South Florida *Sun-Sentinel* dining critic and food columnist

"Sef's enthusiasm, though some would call it madness, about the great American hamburger is contagious. To know him is to participate in it, trust me. And I've found the only thing better than grabbing a burger with Burger Beast himself is diving into his book for a taste of the history behind this iconic sandwich."

—Larry Carrino, Brustman Carrino PR, President

"So you're asking yourself, 'Where did it all begin?' *All about the Burger* is a fun-to-read, witty book with tons of information about everyone's favorite meat in between two buns. It's must-read for all those burger connoisseurs around the world!

—Michell Sanchez, Latin House, chef and owner

"Sef knows comfort food, but not like you and me. Sef wants to know the history of a food, of a place, and how they influenced one another. He takes a scholarly approach to deeply research the history of the most American creation—the hamburger—and makes a meal of it. To a history buff, *All about the Burger* is as satisfying as a bacon double cheeseburger (hold the tomatoes)."

—Carlos Frías, food and dining editor, *Miami Herald*

"HOLY CRAP! That is some education that I just received. So cool..."

**—Adam Feigeles, Adam's Filling Station Food Truck,
chef and owner**

"An insightful look into the world of burgers along with glimpses into the business behind the scenes. A fun read on a subject we can all relate to."

—Scott Savin, Magic City Casino, CEO

"No one knows more about the rise and popularity of all things beef-on-bun—from national hamburger chains to regional specialties—than Sef Gonzalez a.k.a. Burger Beast. He's a treasure, and *All about the Burger* is a must-read for any accomplished eater."

—Evan S. Benn, former *Miami Herald* food editor

"*All about the burger* is an amazing read that took me back in time and brought up some great childhood memories, all while teaching me things I never knew about the places I loved to visit."

—Jimmy Piedrahita, Mojo Donuts & Fried Chicken, owner

"*All about the Burger* is the national story of one of America's favorite foods that is digestible at a local level. Burger Beast shares the unknown and obscure facts that only a passionate historian can uncover."

—Jorge Zamanillo, History Miami Museum,
   Executive Director

"I laughed, I cried, but most of all, *All about the Burger* made me hungry. Don't read *All about the Burger* on an empty stomach... you'll regret it.

"*All about the Burger* is the go-to source for America's tastiest subject. Hats off to Burger Beast for bringing over a hundred years of burger history together for all to enjoy."

—Billy Kramer, NFA Burger, owner

"Sef uncovers details of hamburger history that not only fascinate, but will make the reader hunger for the next chapter."

—David Hosticka, Dog 'n Suds, Muskegon, Michigan
   location owner

"In *All about the Burger*, Burger Beast takes the meat from out of the buns for all to see, an in-detail look at the various soap operas 'novelas' that built our fascination with this hand-held delight. A read and re-read that should be on a reference shelf."

—Barry Hennessey, El Gringo de las Fritas

"*All about the Burger* is certainly packed with information about the great American staple sandwich, and the Burger Beast brings years of great research to the table, painting the picture of how some of our favorite chains came into existence. As a fellow restaurant historian, I find the Beast's knowledge of fast food chains to be second to none, and he has proven to be a tremendous resource in my own quest for knowledge about America's greatest eateries."

—Troy Smith, *Restaurant Rewind* YouTube channel

"*All about the Burger* tells the complex story of a simple meal. Who knew that the history of the hamburger was fraught with all the elements that would make for an unexpectedly dynamic read? ...The Burger Beast. That's who!"
—Paul Hernandez , City of Hialeah Councilman

" 'Where's the beef?' If there's one person who knows the beef's whereabouts and how it got there, it is Sef 'The Burger Beast' Gonzalez, and he'll tell you all about it in *All about the Burger*. With an inside look at the national burger scenes, burger competitions, and specialty burgers—including an entire chapter dedicated to the Frita Cubana! The Beast gives burger lovers the cheese on the birth and evolution of one of the most enduring cultural and culinary American phenomenon."
—Ivonne B. Ward

"A must-read for anyone who agrees that the burger is one of the most iconic foods in America. This book has been painstakingly researched with so many details and inside information that will satisfy the cravings of any burger aficionado. With all of the craft burgers we have available now, this book gives us a historical view on how this American food staple became so prominent in our culture."
—Adrian Simo

"The Burger Beast is tapped into the main line of South Florida burger culture. Hamburger aficionados will be fascinated by the Beast's collection of burger lore."
—JC Lopez

"This is exactly like eating fries out of the drive-thru bag. The next bit of history is better than the last and leaves you wanting more of that salty goodness."
—**Charlie Calderin**

"Burgers, history, business, and great stories! Love it. We drive by these places every day and sometimes we take them for granted. Thanks for sharing the stories of these visionaries with us Burger Beast."
—**Javier De La Vega**

"If you love food and consider yourself a foodie, then this is the book for you. Burger Beast's attention to detail is second to none. Beast has a real passion for telling the history of the burger. Run, don't walk to get many copies of this book, and give them to your friends, especially the vegan ones."
—**Dan Vezina**

all about

the

BURGER

Published by Mango Publishing Group, a division of Mango Media Inc.

Cover, Layout & Design: Morgane Leoni
Author Picture: Copyright © Al Diaz

For permission requests, please contact the publisher at:
Mango Publishing Group
2850 S Douglas Road, 2nd Floor
Coral Gables, FL 33134 USA
info@mango.bz

For special orders, quantity sales, course adoptions and corporate sales, please email the publisher at sales@mango.bz. For trade and wholesale sales, please contact Ingram Publisher Services at:
customer.service@ingramcontent.com or +1.800.509.4887.

All About the Burger: A History of America's Favorite Sandwich

Library of Congress Cataloging-in-Publication number: 2019932091
ISBN: (print) 978-1-63353-962-4, (ebook) 978-1-63353-963-1
BISAC category code HIS054000 HISTORY / Social History

Printed in the United States of America

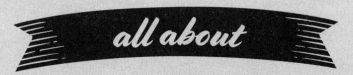

all about

the

BURGER

A HISTORY OF AMERICA'S FAVORITE SANDWICH

Sef "Burger Beast" Gonzalez

Mango Publishing

CORAL GABLES, FL

To my parents, Cary and Serafin,
for everything you selflessly do.

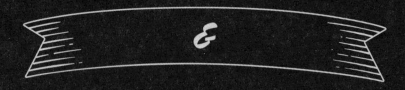

&

To my wife, Marcela, there could be no
Beast without his Beauty.

INGREDIENTS

Foreword

As a rule, I trust very few people. And when it comes to burger knowledge, I trust even fewer. I've spent the better part of the last twenty years researching, eating, thinking, writing, talking about, and generally loving hamburgers. In those years, I have taken the deep dive into the truth about the American hamburger and why we love them so. In many cases, I have spent far too much time trying to get it right and can barely count on two hands my truest burger allies. But when I met Sef Gonzalez, I realized I was in the presence of someone I could trust.

I was struck by his dedication to the Burgerverse, and we became instant friends and confidantes. In the past decade, we've regularly traded findings on burger joints and speak often about the poorly documented history of the American hamburger. And just when I think I've got a certain history or timeline correct, Sef is there with a new detail. On more occasions than I'd like to admit, usually immediately following an Instagram post or a mention in a newspaper, Sef has set me straight. Sef is deeply knowledgeable about many of the burgerways in America, and for this I'm constantly grateful.

When he told me he was considering opening The Burger Museum to house his growing collection of burger ephemera, I thought, *Who better?* followed by. *How much stuff could he have?* In my mind, it was sure to be a cute one-room pocket museum with a few cool items. When I first set foot in the place, I was knocked over by the more than 3,500 items on display, many one-of-a-kind. A new level of appreciation had been achieved.

To me, the hamburger is one of the greatest gastronomic expressions of American proletarian food with its rich and varied history. Sef has done his research, and this book is arguably the definitive resource on a subject very dear to the both of us. Lose yourself in the stories which make up the patchwork that is the fabric of America, and learn why after more than a century, we love burgers today more than ever.

GEORGE MOTZ

Professor of Hamburgers at NYU,

Brooklyn, 2019

Introduction

Before we get started, let's set one important ground rule here. I'll only be talking about hamburgers. In my world, ground beef in patty form cooked and placed between bread is a hamburger sandwich. Yes...sandwich. I said it once, and I'll be saying it again throughout the book. The hamburger is a sandwich—always has been and always will be.

I have loved hamburgers since as far back as I can remember. My earliest burger recollections are with my mother, Cary, when she worked in Miami Beach. Mom would wait to take her lunch break with my dad, Serafin; my sister, Michelle; and me. We would then head out to McDonald's. There were no golden arches near our home, so this was a rare treat. I always ate a burger with minced onions, cheese, ketchup, and mustard.

The truth is, I was more of a Burger King kid. Miami happens to be BK's hometown, which I'm sure was a contributing factor to their having been the dominant burger restaurant all over South Florida during the 1960s and 1970s.

On Saturdays, my mom would take us through the BK drive-thru after a long day of shopping. The regular cheeseburger was topped with mustard, ketchup, cheese, and those pesky pickles, which I always removed. I had an emotional attachment to this charbroiled burger. It reminded me of the ones my dad would make us on special occasions. And by special occasion, I mean whenever he busted out his BBQ grill.

By the time Wendy's arrived in my neighborhood in the early 1980s, I was in full-bloom burger obsession. Unfortunately, my family had to deal with it. Wendy's happened to be across the street from the printing shop my grandfather owned. He received many an after-school call from me; I would beg him to bring me a single with cheese.

I was bad and some might say out of control. It was around this time that my restaurant ordering habits changed. It didn't matter what type of eatery it was as long as the menu had a burger on it.

Even as I grew older, my love for burgers never left me. A little over ten years ago, my life drastically changed course after many years spent in retail management. I needed an outlet to destress after long days of dealing with customers. My wife, Marcela, suggested I write a blog about my love for burgers. When I couldn't come up with a suitable name, she said, "Burger Beast!" I was like, "Huh?!" Yes, my friends, my wife believed that I ate my burgers like a beast, and so my *nom de plume* was born.

The *Burger Beast* blog, along with my social media posts, still chronicles my visits to all types of restaurants. However, there is a focus on mom-and-pop establishments that sell burgers and comfort food. Any historical background on the spots where I have eaten is eventually added to my musings.

My friend "Bulldog" Jim Winters ended up gifting me an old Burger Chef sign. At first, I wasn't familiar with Burger Chef, but within a week I was well versed in it. The burger steward side of me had been awakened.

I now remember it as if it all happened overnight. It really didn't though. There were bins and bins of memorabilia from all of my online purchases hidden away in my old bedroom at my parent's house. My yearly road trips had begun to include stops at old-school burger joints. Antique shops and anywhere I could do some picking helped grow my collection.

It wasn't long before my mom strongly suggested I find a new home for everything. She was over my using my old sleeping grounds as a storage facility.

The old Burger Beast headquarters became home to three rooms decorated with parts of the collection. It was during a meeting at our

HQ that Scott Savin, CEO of Miami's Magic City Casino, saw my collection. A few days later, I pitched the idea of having MCC lease me some space at the casino. They said yes, and a full-fledged Burger Museum opened in December 2016.

I've been lucky enough to meet hundreds of burger lovers from across the world at my Burger Museum. I love it when they tell me about what great memories the collection stirs for them. Plus, I'm able to have discussions with them about their favorites and find out facts that I never knew. The Burger Museum has been a great learning experience for me. It has only deepened my love for all things burger.

All about the Burger is the next logical step in my burger evolution. For posterity's sake, I had been documenting little details and stories that hadn't made it into other great books about burgers. My own book is the ideal vehicle in which to share them.

I will take you through every era of the burger movement. We'll talk about little-known historical facts, regional burger specialties, the Burger Wars, burger festivals, and much more.

It is also crucial that those restaurants which helped shape our love for burgers, as well as their individual histories, are well represented. Whenever applicable, any innovations are covered as well.

At this point all I'm doing is holding you up. Go forward and read, my friend.

Chapter

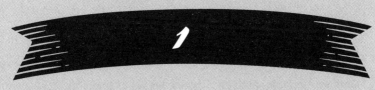

1

THE BEGINNING

There is no set-in-stone, 100 percent accurate history of how the hamburger came to be in the United States.

It is believed, however, that its origins go back to the Mongols, who would ride with minced meat stored under their horse saddles. The theory was that the meat (mutton) would be tenderized during their long rides. After the Mongols invaded Russia in the 1200s, bringing their minced meat with them, the Russians adopted it and made it a part of their cuisine as "steak tartare."

During the fifteenth century, steak tartare was introduced to the Germans, who would eventually shape and refine the delicacy. The dish made its way to New York in the nineteenth century from the port of Hamburg, Germany, and then became known as Hamburg Steak. By the way, Hamburger in German means "from Hamburg," just as Frankfurter means "from Frankfurt."

It began popping up on US menus, but the first recorded use of the term "Hamburg Steak" didn't happen until the 1880s. In 1887, the *Chicago Tribune* mentioned that Hamburg Steak was "made by chopping any lean piece of beef and cooking it with onions or garlic." The first time the word "Hamburger" made an appearance was in the *Walla Walla Union*, a newspaper in the state of Washington, in an article on January 5, 1889.

I thought you might get a kick out of some of the quotes I found with the word hamburger in them.

HAMBURGERS IN THE NEWS

1893
"Fraker's celebrated Hamburger steak sandwiches are always on hand to replenish an empty stomach and even fortify Satan himself."
—*Evening Gazette* **(Reno, Nevada)**

1895
"Mike's face looked like a Hamburger sandwich."
—*Washington Times* **(Washington, District of Columbia)**

1896
"A distinguished favorite, only five cents, is Hamburger steak sandwich, the meat for which is kept ready in small patties and cooked while you wait on the gasoline range."
—*Chicago Tribune* **(Chicago, Illinois)**

1897
"He was very drunk and knocked a hamburger sandwich out of her hand."
—*St. Louis-Post Dispatch* **(St. Louis, Missouri)**

1905
"Try a hamburger steak sandwich at Worsham & Zook's"
—*Chariton Courier* **(Keytesville, Missouri)**

1906
"Harris was cooking a hamburger steak sandwich for a hungry car conductor who had come in from a run and was deftly flopping the steak on its other side, when leakage from the gasoline stove tank became ignited and exploded."
—*Buffalo Courier* **(Buffalo, New York)**

1907

"Don't forget that we are the people that can satisfy your hunger with an Oyster Stew, or a Bowl of Chile, or a good old Hamburger Sandwich. We also have one of the choicest lines of fine cigars in town"

—**LA Reinecke, The Owl Cafe; in** *The Louisburg Herald* **(Louisburg, Kansas)**

1909

"Fort Scott People Are Turning into Hamburg Sandwich Fiends"

—**Headline,** *Fort Scott Tribune-Monitor* **(Fort Scott, Kansas)**

1910

"D.H. Culmer is recovering from a severe attack of ptomaine poisoning. He ate a hamburger steak sandwich at a restaurant and was soon taken with convulsions, suffering extremely. Several men were required to hold him. A physician worked with him for four hours, after which he was removed to his home from the grocery store of C.E. Payne, where he is employed"

—*Evening Times-Republican* **(Marshalltown, Iowa)**

1911

"S.R. Maxson Has the ONLY place to get a nice cup of coffee or hot hamburger sandwich."

—*The Argos Reflector* **(Argos, Indiana)**

1911
"Perhaps the oddest bit of evidence ever filed in a Court of Justice was a hamburger sandwich, turned over today to Prosecutor Burns from the Justice's Court of Harry Hughes, in the case of the State of Ohio against Tom Buzanik, recently fined thirty-five dollars for the alleged mixing of salt of sulphur in this hamburger meat, in order to give it a rich appearance. Buzanik appealed the case. The hamburger sandwich is now several weeks old, and its odor is strengthening with age."
—*The Cincinnati Enquirer* **(Cincinnati, Ohio)**

1918
"Hot Hamburger Steak Sandwich with Brown Gravy from Statler's Lunch—twenty cents"
—*The Buffalo Times* **(Buffalo, New York)**

1919
"Hamburger Steak Sandwich from Kresge's five and ten Store—five cents"
—*St. Louis Post-Dispatch* **(St. Louis Missouri)**

DID YOU KNOW?

In 1918, "Liberty Steak" would become a common replacement for the word hamburger steak. Americans were getting out of World War I, and with patriotism on a high, the use of a German word was not going to fly. Later on, during World War II at the 1941 National Association of Retail Meat Merchants, butchers agreed to change the name of hamburgers to "defense steak." Much like liberty steak before it, defense steak was in use for a few years before it disappeared altogether.

WHO MADE THE FIRST HAMBURGER?

There are many claims to the creation of the first hamburger. Here are four that I believe are the best of the bunch.

Hamburger Charlie

In 1885, Charles "Hamburger Charlie" Nagreen traveled to Seymour, Wisconsin, in his ox-driven cart with 1,500 feet of lumber inside to build a meatball stand at the Outagamie County Fair. He was only fifteen years old at the time. He realized the attendees weren't going to be able to walk around, enjoy the exhibits, and eat a meatball all at the same time, making his original idea a bust. So Nagreen smashed a meatball and sandwiched it between two pieces of bread. This was a success, and he returned to sell hamburgers at this fair every year. He passed away on June 5, 1951.

On August 6, 2005, a fourteen-foot tall statue of Hamburger Charlie was unveiled at the seventeenth annual Burger Fest in Seymour. There is a plaque with "Charlie's Chant" located at the base of the statue:

"Hamburger, hamburger, hamburger hot, with an onion in the middle and a pickle on top, makes your lips go flippity-flop, come on over, try an order, fried in butter, listen to it sputter."

A few years later, the Wisconsin Legislature proclaimed Charles Nagreen as the inventor of the hamburger and Seymour as the "Home of the Hamburger."

The Menches Family

Frank and Charles Menches were traveling concessionaires in 1885–1892. They customarily sold ground sausage sandwiches but were running low on product. After a trip to the butcher showed they only had ground beef available, they changed the protein in their sandwich. It tasted bland, so they added brown sugar, coffee, and a few other ingredients to liven it up.

In an October 4, 1951, obituary in the *Akron Beacon Journal* titled, "Frank Menches Dies, Invented Hamburger," it states that this all happened on the opening day of the Summit County Fair in 1892. The article also mentions that two years later at the Elyria Fair, Frank named it the hamburger.

But the Menches family maintains that this all took place in 1885 at the Erie County Fair in Hamburg, New York. They said that when someone asked what the sandwich was called, Frank looked up and saw the banner for the festival and said, "This is the hamburger." In this version, the name for the sandwich is derived from the city in which it was first served, not Hamburg, Germany.

In 1991, the great-grandchildren of Charles Menches discovered a copy of the original recipe. They followed the path set forth by their burger ancestors by selling the hamburgers at fairs, and this eventually led to the opening of the first Menches Brother restaurant in Green, Ohio, on March 7, 1994. It has since closed. Currently, the family owns restaurants in Canton, Massillon, and Uniontown, Ohio.

The brothers also lay claim to inventing the ice cream cone at the 1904 St. Louis World's Fair.

Louis' Lunch

Louis' Lunch in New Haven, Connecticut, claims that Louis Lassen is not only responsible for the hamburger, but the steak sandwich, too.

What we do know is that in 1900, Louis took some of the leftover trimmings used for his steak sandwich, ground them up, and placed them between two slices of toast. He served this hamburger sandwich from his lunch cart to a customer who was on the go. Years later, the legendary meat wagon was retired when he moved into a space with indoor seating.

In July 2000, the Library of Congress acknowledged Louis Lassen as the creator of the hamburger and Louis' Lunch as the location where the first hamburger was served. The first steak sandwich was also acknowledged as a Louis' Lunch first.

The documentation submitted to the Library of Congress included a history of Louis' Lunch, magazine and newspaper articles, photographs, and a personal account written by Kenneth Lassen, Louis' grandson.

You can still enjoy one of Louis' famous hamburgers; the fifth generation of Lassens now runs Louis' Lunch. The burgers come with cheese spread, tomato, and onion.

Fletcher Davis

Texas historian Frank X. Tolbert said in 1979 that Fletcher "Uncle Fletch" Davis was the inventor of the hamburger. He even hosted a contest to celebrate its seventy-fifth anniversary, claiming that the hamburger was introduced at the World's Fair in 1904. The original burger, said Tolbert, was a half-pound beef patty on a toasted bun with mustard, lettuce, tomato, and onions.

In November, 2006, Texas state representative Betty Brown asked the Texas Legislature to "formally designate" Athens, Texas, as the "Original Home of the Hamburger." This designation is based on Fletcher Davis's lunch counter, where he sold meat sandwiches in Athens sometime in the late 1800s. On March 22, 2007, the resolution was passed.

We will probably never know exactly who came up with the hamburger that we all love so much. I do have a quote from the *Indianapolis Star* in November of 1964 that is a perfect segue to the next chapter.

> For many years a so-called hamburger sandwich had been sold at fairs, amusement parks, carnivals, and in some restaurants. These sandwiches were prepared by placing a thick patty of ground beef on a griddle or skillet, allowing it to cook over a slow fire for an indefinite time, and placing it in a cold bun. The meat in this sandwich was practically tasteless, as most of the valuable juices and nutriment had been cooked out of it.
>
> —Billy Ingram, Cofounder of White Castle

Chapter

2

WHITE CASTLE

Who would have thought that a five-stool burger stand in Wichita, Kansas, would be responsible for changing the course of hamburger history?

Walter Anderson, who had owned and operated many restaurants, got the ball rolling. He created a unique method of preparing the hamburger. It involved smashing the beef patty, along with some shredded onions, with a spatula, then turning it over and placing both halves of the bun on the meat to pick up the steam and flavors. Across the street from the hamburger stand where he worked was a remodeled street car, now home to a shoe shop.

On October 16, 1916, after purchasing the street car for sixty dollars (almost $1,500 today), he installed three stools and a counter that he built, along with an icebox. His small budget left him with enough money to buy a flat piece of iron that would act as a flat-top. It wasn't the ideal situation for cooking hamburgers because the grease would drip off the edges, but he made do. He also ground and prepared the meat directly behind the counter, which helped dispel the public's uneasiness about eating ground beef.

Outside of his hamburger stand, he hung a sign that read "Hamburgers 5¢." Anderson made $3.75 in sales on that first day. He launched the catchphrase, "Buy 'em by the Sack," to encourage customers to buy his burgers by the half dozen.

WALTER MEETS BILLY

Anderson's first location proved to be successful, and by 1920 he had added two more stands. Around this time, he met Edgar Waldo "Billy"

Ingram, a real estate broker and insurance salesman. Ingram also helped Anderson get the lease for his third location. It was when Anderson attempted to get a lease for a fourth location that some issues arose, and Billy intervened. This new partnership was called White Castle, a name was chosen by Billy, who said that *White* stood for purity and cleanliness, while *Castle* represented strength, permanence, and stability.

To get the first stand open, they borrowed seven hundred dollars in bond money, which they paid back in about ninety days. In 1926, the cost to open a burger stand was $3,500, or about fifty thousand dollars today. The first White Castle building had only five stools, measured fifteen by ten feet, and was made of cement blocks. It opened at 110 West First Street in Wichita, Kansas, on March 21, 1921.

White Castle was such a hit that by the end of 1921, copycat restaurants started to pop up.

These stands not only sold hamburgers but used a variation of the "Buy 'em by the Sack" catchphrase. A few straight-up used, copied, or were inspired by White Castle architecture. The best known were Kewpee Hotel Hamburgs (Flint, Michigan), The Krystal (Chattanooga, Tennessee), Little Tavern (Louisville, Kentucky), Maid-Rite (Muscatine, Iowa), Royal Castle (Miami, Florida), and White Tower (Milwaukee, Wisconsin).

Even the cities where White Castle opened faced the same issue. Once they established themselves, new competition would show up. Indianapolis was different. A former employee opened a shop there before White Castle had even arrived.

WHITE CASTLE INNOVATES

Billy Ingram started to differentiate White Castle from everyone else through innovation, pioneering new methods and ideas:

Better spatulas

Pancake turners were used to cook hamburgers, but they were not made to stand up to the job. So they cut old saws into pieces that were roughly about two inches square, then soldered a handle to make a custom spatula. Eventually, they found a manufacturer.

Electric dishwashers

White Castle was one of the first to install under-the-counter electric dishwashers. These forced them to redesign their mugs so that the rinse water would drain through slots on their bottom rims.

Better exhaust systems

Billy created an exhaust system that allowed the fumes from the hot flat-top to escape upwards via an enamel hood and later a glass hood.

Improved meat sources

As they expanded into new cities, White Castle would locate a meat supplier that only used US government-inspected beef from specific cuts to give it the right flavor.

Paper hats

They procured a patent for folded-paper hats to replace the linen ones of the day. Four years later, as the Paperlynen Company, they manufactured paper hats not only for themselves, but for other restaurants.

Custom buns

White Castle had two bakeries making all of their buns.

Special cartons

A cardboard carton with heat lining was created (the first of its kind in the food industry) so that the burgers at the bottom of the sack would not get soggy or crushed.

000

In 1924, the company transitioned from partnership status to incorporating as the White Castle System of Eating House Corporation. The following year, they opened their twentieth location.

To encourage closer relationships between the home office and its employees, plus customers who might be interested, Billy Ingram created a company newsletter named the *Hot Hamburger*. The name was later switched to *The White Castle Official House Organ* after a December 1925 contest.

The creation and patenting of a moveable, all-metal White Castle building design with enamel panels on the outside happened in 1928. Due to constant design changes in their early days, fifty-five of them were built. Six years later, White Castle created a new division, Porcelain Steel Buildings Company, to fabricate their castles and equipment.

The switch to frozen beef from fresh happened in 1931 when one of the larger meatpacking companies was able to ship square frozen beef patties to anywhere that White Castle wanted. As they rolled out the frozen patty program over the next few years, it also helped to standardize the hamburgers at every restaurant.

ADVERTISING WORKS

June 3, 1932, was a historic day for the company. They ran a "buy two, get three for free" coupon ad in the local newspaper for the following day at three in the afternoon. Some experts in the marketing field told them that very few, if any, customers would be interested in using a coupon for a free hamburger. By two o'clock the next day, most of their locations had lines of eager hamburger consumers ready to cash in their coupons. It was such a challenge to keep up with the demand that the next time the ad ran, it was good for five to seven days instead of just one.

Another ingenious idea was a program White Castle created to educate mothers and homemakers about the sanitary conditions of their restaurants and the quality of their food. There was a "Julia Joyce" in every city who would act as the company hostess and guide the ladies around their local White Castles. Upon the completion of the tour, the women were presented with one coupon for five carryout hamburgers for ten cents, and another coupon valid the following Saturday for hamburgers for children.

BILLY GOES IT ALONE

In 1933, Walter Anderson sold out all his interests in White Castle to Billy Ingram for $340,000. The following year, Billy decided to move all company operations from Wichita to a more centralized location at 555 Goodale Street in Columbus, Ohio. The White Castle general offices, along with the Paperlynen Company and the new Porcelain Steel Buildings Company divisions, would have homes there.

By April 1933, White Castles were in 125 locations in sixteen different cities. The mid-1930s found White Castle adding carhop service to their restaurants to compete with the growing drive-in culture. Curb service ended in 1972, as drive-thrus were now the next big thing.

During World War II, Porcelain Steel Buildings Company was not allowed to produce anything that did not support the war, so they accepted contracts to build amphibious vehicles. Meanwhile, the White Castle locations had to deal with meat rationing by selling whatever they had available to them.

"If we had some ham, we could have some ham and eggs—if we had some eggs," said Billy Ingram in 1943. "If we had enough help, we could do a good business—if we had something to sell."

WHITE CASTLE SLIDERS EVOLVE

In 1943, there was a significant change in White Castle cooking technique as Billy Ingram visited every Castle. Dehydrated onions were laid out all over the griddle, and the burger patties were placed on top of them. The buns then covered the patties and onions. This method minimized waste from flipping, which tended to break patties, and shortened the cooking time. By the time rationing ended in 1946, the price of a hamburger was ten cents, double what it had been just seven years earlier.

Between 1949 and 1953, White Castle developed a new hamburger patty with five holes in it. The new patty sped up cooking times with a new steam grilled technique. It also steamed the buns better. The idea was so great that they took out a patent on it.

As the economy began bouncing back in the 1950s, White Castle expanded into high-traffic cities like Detroit, Cleveland, Miami, and New York.

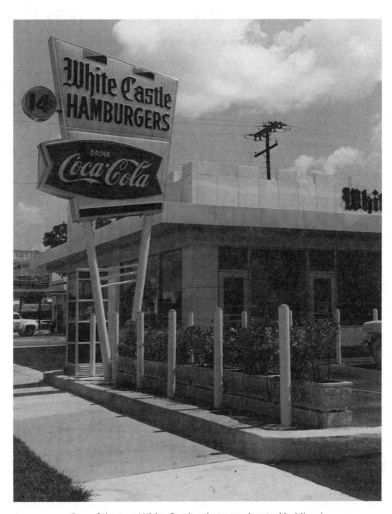

One of the two White Castles that were located in Miami, Florida. The restaurants opened in early 1959 after Billy Ingram retired there.

HOME IS WHERE THE BURGER IS

During this period, customers who longed for White Castle hamburgers could now buy frozen patties and ship them to their homes. This led to the creation of a White Castle frozen food division in 1987, selling burgers to supermarkets across the US and helping people like me fulfill my long-distance cravings.

WHITE CASTLE'S CONTEMPORARIES PROFILES

In chronological order.

Kewpee Hotel Hamburgs

Year Founded: *1923*
City Founded: *Flint, Michigan*
Founder: *Samuel V. Blair*
Number of Locations at the Chain's Peak: *over 400*
Slogans: *"Mity Nice Hamburger," "Your Granpappy ate here!"* and *"Hamburg pickle on top, makes your heart go flippity-flop!"*

▶ Kewpee was one of the first drive-in restaurants.

▶ In 1958, Bill Thomas purchased the Kewpee franchise in Flint, Michigan. Due to a trademark dispute in 1967, he switched the name to Bill Thomas' Halo Burger. As of 2019, Halo Burger has ten locations operating in Genesee County, Michigan.

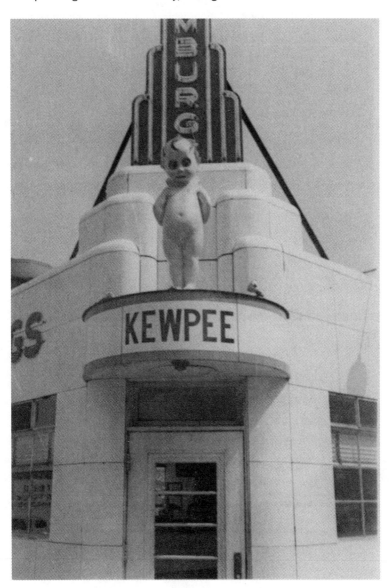

Entry door along to Kewpee Hotel Hamburgs in the 1930s
with large Kewpie doll looking down.

▶ In 1963, the Grand Rapids, Michigan, franchisees broke away as Mr. Fables. The name Mr. Fables came from the founding cousins' surnames, Dick Faber and John Boyles. Mr. Fables closed up shop in 2000, twelve years after the founders sold the company.

▶ In his autobiography, Dave Thomas, founder of Wendy's, said that Kewpee was an inspiration to him. He frequented the location in Kalamazoo, Michigan, when he was a child.

▶ After being approved for listing on the National Register of Historic Places, the downtown Lima Kewpee location never made the list. The reason? The final application had "Owner Objection" stamped on it.

▶ There are three Kewpees in Lima, Ohio; one in Lansing, Michigan; and another in Racine, Wisconsin; all still open for business.

Maid-Rite

Year Founded: *1926*
City Founded: *Muscatine, Iowa*
Founder: *Fred Angell*
Number of Locations at the Chain's Peak: *between 300 and 400*
Slogan: *"We Do It Rite!"*

▶ While technically not hamburgers, Maid-Rite's loose meat sandwiches are very close cousins. They're made up of ground beef and spices served on a hamburger roll.

▶ The original Maid-Rite sandwich came with pickles, mustard, and onion.

▶ The Maid-Rite Sandwich Shop in Springfield, Illinois, predates the Maid-Rite company by two years. Since 1984, this location's building has been a part of the National Register of Historic Places. They also claim to have the first drive-thru window in the US.

▶ The Maid-Rite company has over thirty restaurants located in Iowa, Illinois, Minnesota, Missouri, and Ohio, not counting a few former franchisees.

White Tower

Founded: *November 17, 1926*
City Founded: *Milwaukee, Wisconsin*
Founders: *John E. Saxe, Thomas E. Saxe*
Number of Locations at the Chain's Peak: *over 230*
Slogans: *"Buy a Bagful"* and *"Take Home a Bagful"*

▶ White Tower restaurants patterned themselves after White Castle. The founders thoroughly investigated White Castle, going so far as to hire a former White Castle operator before opening the first White Tower restaurant. All of this came out over the course of two lawsuits, one of which was brought in 1929 in Minnesota by White Castle against White Tower. White Tower then counter-sued in a Michigan court claiming that they had arrived in Michigan first. The 1930 Minnesota court ruling found in favor of White Castle, forcing White Tower to end all use of their similar name, architecture, and slogans.

▶ While White Castle did not force White Tower to change their name as per the ruling, they were required to pay a onetime licensing fee for its use to the tune of eighty-two thousand dollars.

ALL ABOUT THE BURGER

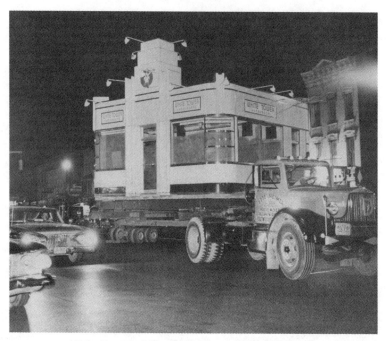

White Tower building moving from Washington Ave to
Central Ave in New York on October 23, 1962.

- White Tower hamburgers weighed one ounce and were served on a two-inch wide roll.

- The Towerettes were White Tower employees who were dressed as nurses to promote the sanitary motif associated with the "White" in their name.

- White Tower tested a "Tower-O-Matic" automated restaurant concept during the 1950s and 1960s that proved to be unsuccessful.

- White Tower locations were slowly sold off, city by city, during the 1980s, until the early 1990s when its parent company left the restaurant business altogether.

- The Tombrock Corporation, formerly known as the White Tower Management Corporation, still exists as a real estate investment and management company based out of New Canaan, Connecticut.

- There is one independently owned White Tower restaurant still open in Toledo, Ohio.

Little Tavern

> Year Founded: *1927*
> City Founded: *Louisville, Kentucky*
> Founder: *Harry F. Duncan*
> Number of Locations at the Chain's Peak: *almost 50*
> Slogan: *"Buy 'em by the bag!"*

- During their first few years of operation, the buildings resembled White Castles of the era.

- The third Little Tavern location in Baltimore opened on January 29, 1931. The Tudor-style building that housed its debut at this location would be the signature look for all future Little Tavern structures.

- In Laurel, Maryland, you will find the last Little Tavern. It reopened in 2008 as Little Tavern Donuts after having been in operation for sixty-six years, then closing in 2006. The original recipe for the burgers is on the menu.

The Krystal

Year Founded: *1932*
City: *Chattanooga, Tennessee*
Founders: *Rody Davenport Jr., J. Glenn Sherrill*
Number of Locations at the Chain's Peak: *420*
Original Slogan: *"Take Along a Sack Full"*

▸ Krystal's first customer was French Jenkins, who spent thirty-five cents on six Krystals (their signature slider) and a cup of coffee.

▸ Company lore says that Davenport's wife suggested the name of crystal with a 'K' after having seen a crystal ball lawn ornament. Krystal's restaurants have often sported a crystal ball on the roof top.

▸ The Krystal Square Off was an event sanctioned by the former International Federation of Competitive Eating (now called Major League Eating) held from 2004 to 2009. Contestants had to eat as many Krystal hamburgers in eight minutes as possible. Joey Chestnut set the current world record on October 28, 2007, with 103 Krystal hamburgers.

▸ In a 2017 interview, Priscilla Presley mentioned that while in Memphis, Tennessee, Elvis Presley loved to eat Krystal hamburgers.

▸ Krystal and White Castle's locations only overlap in Kentucky (Bowling Green, London, and Somerset) and in Nashville, Tennessee.

▸ Krystal currently operates over three hundred sixty restaurants in Alabama, Arkansas, Florida, Georgia, Kentucky, Louisiana, Mississippi, North Carolina, South Carolina, Tennessee, and Virginia.

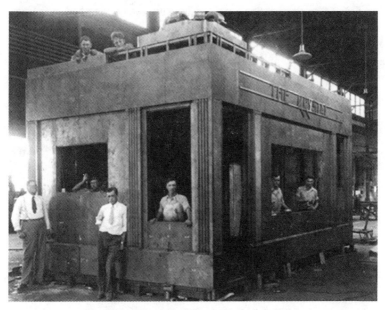

The original Krystal building being built in 1931. It was manufactured in Chicago then brought down to Chattanooga.

Steak 'n Shake

Year Founded: *1934*
City: *Normal, Illinois*
Founders: *Augustus "Gus" Hamilton Belt, Edith L. Belt*
Number of Locations at the Chain's Peak: *more than 577*
Original Slogan: *"In Sight It Must Be Right"* and *"Tak-Homa-Sak"*

- Gus Belt owned the Shell Inn, a combination gas station and restaurant. He borrowed three hundred dollars against the furniture in his apartment from a bank to fix up the building.

- "I'm going to start a drive-in. I'm going to have the finest hamburger in the country and a real, honest-to-goodness milkshake. Customers can come up, park, and get waited on in the car. Or they can eat at a counter inside." Gus said to his friend Hynie Johnson, a sign painter. The going rate for a hamburger at the time was five cents, and he planned to sell his at ten cents.

- When the first location opened in February 1934, it could serve up to fifty customers inside.

- It was called "Whitehouse Steak 'n Shake" after the popular "white house" restaurant style. The Whitehouse surname was dropped since everyone referred to them as Steak n Shake.

- When Steak 'n Shake had three locations, Gus Belt had a habit of wheeling in a barrel of T-bone, sirloin, and round steaks and then grinding them up into steakburgers right in front of his customers. The idea was to show them what went into their burgers, hence the slogan "In Sight It Must Be Right."

- The Rocky Mountain Hamburger Company from Denver had "Tak-Homa-Sak" on their wall. The president gave Gus Belt permission to use it for Steak 'n Shake.

- When World War II caused beef shortages, Gus Belt took it into his own hands to make sure that Steak 'n Shake would not be affected. He purchased a farm and bootlegged cattle to make sure that his fifteen locations had could serve their steakburgers.

- The Steak 'n Shake on Route 66 at Springfield, Missouri, was built in 1962 and made the National Register of Historic Places in 2012.

- Today, there are 577 Steak 'n Shakes worldwide in Alabama, Arizona, Arkansas, California, Colorado, Florida, Georgia, Illinois, Indiana, Iowa, Kansas, Kentucky, Louisiana, Michigan, Mississippi, Missouri, Nevada, New Jersey, North Carolina, Ohio, Oklahoma, Pennsylvania, South Carolina, Tennessee, Texas, Utah, Virginia, Washington, West Virginia, and outside the US in France, Italy, Kuwait, Portugal, Qatar, Saudi Arabia, Spain, and the United Kingdom.

Wimpy Grills

Year Founded: *1934*
City: *Bloomington, Indiana*
Founder: *Edward Gold*
Number of Locations at the Chain's Peak: *over 1,500 worldwide*
Original Slogan: *"The Glorified Hamburger"*

- The character of J. Wellington Wimpy from the Popeye cartoon series was the inspiration for the Wimpy Grills name.

- Wimpy Grills were closely associated with Chicago, Illinois, but did not open their first location there until 1936. The number of Wimpy Grill restaurants in Chicago grew to twenty-six in 1947.

- In 1954, Edward Gold licensed the use of the name to J. Lyons and Co. for an expansion in the United Kingdom. Three years later, he partnered with J. Lyons and Co to create Wimpy's International, which grew to more than 1,500 locations. Gold later sold his shares in the partnership to Lyons.

- 1967 saw the first South African Wimpy location open in Durban. The South African restaurants were spun off and sold in the late 1970s. Famous Brands Limited acquired those locations in 2003, and then in 2007, acquired the Wimpy International Ltd. company.

- By the time of the founder's death in 1977, the number of locations in the US had dwindled to nine. No one purchased the businesses and trademark upon his passing, so Wimpy's disappeared from the US burger scene.

- Today, there are almost seventy restaurants in operation in the United Kingdom and nearly five hundred in South Africa.

Royal Castle

Year Founded: *1938 in Miami, 1940 in Cleveland*
City: *Miami, Florida*
Founder: *William Singer*
Number of Locations at the Chain's Peak: *more than 200*
Original Slogan: *"Fit for a King!"*

- Many folks are familiar with the Royal Castle based out of Miami, which expanded to Georgia and Louisiana, but did not know there was a separate Royal Castle company operating in Cleveland, Ohio, run by William Singer's brother Samuel.

- During its opening week of sales in Miami, the first store grossed $245.

- Upon entering most Royal Castles, you would find the Royal Castle "Fit for a King" slogan embedded in the terrazzo floor.

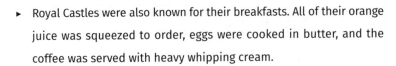

- Royal Castles were also known for their breakfasts. All of their orange juice was squeezed to order, eggs were cooked in butter, and the coffee was served with heavy whipping cream.

- Royal Castle ended up bottling their famous house-made Birch Beer and selling it in Florida supermarkets.

- When he worked for Prince Castle, Ray Kroc of McDonald's fame sold multimixer shake machines to Royal Castle.

- In an effort to compete with the speed at which McDonald's and their contemporaries could pump out burgers, Royal Castle began making the burgers in advance. The burgers would sit in a holding drawer, which affected the quality and taste.

- Royal Castle sold the company to Performance Systems Inc., owners of Minnie Pearl Chicken, in February 1969. Performance Systems then became embroiled in a scandal with the Securities and Trade Commission over their method of reporting franchise fees. By the time that Performance Systems announced 1969 earnings as a loss of thirty-nine million in September 1970, they were in significant financial trouble. Performance Systems was forced to sell Royal Castle locations where the property value far exceeded the profit generated by the restaurant.

- Royal Castle tried to diversify with Royal Carousel, an automated restaurant; Royal Sky Campgrounds; Criterion I Steakhouses; and Pizza Garden. None of them worked. The company attempted to rebrand and change the menu, but it was too late. In 1975, Royal Castle's stockholders began to liquidate the company's assets. The final liquidation payment came in October 1979.

- The 2017 Best Picture Oscar winner *Moonlight* had a scene filmed in the last operating Royal Castle in Miami.

Grand Opening ad for Royal Castle from *The Miami Herald* on March 18, 1938.

The Original Slider Recipe

Four to an order.

INGREDIENTS

- 4 two-ounce balls of 80/20 chuck
- 1 yellow onion, cut thin on a mandoline
- 4 slices American cheese
- 4 smallish rolls
- Kosher salt
- Dill pickles
- Yellow mustard

DIRECTIONS

1. Grab the two-ounce balls of 80/20 ground beef and place them onto the flat-top/griddle.

2. Place thin onions on each ball, then smash into flat-top/griddle until each resembles a beautifully deformed burger patty.

3. Add salt as you would to any burger.

4. After cooking a little bit, flip the burger so the onions end up on the bottom towards the heat surface.

5. As the burger is approaching medium-well done, place a slice of American cheese on it.

6. Then place the bottom bun on the burger, followed by the top one. This technique steams the buns.

7. When the onions turn light brownish, the burger is ready.

8. Set aside top bun for a second.

9. Flip the burger with a spatula with the bottom bun on so the cheese is now on the bottom and the browned onions on top.

10. Add a couple of slices of pickle and a dollop of yellow mustard.

11. Place the top bun on the slider.

12. Now you eat!

Chapter

3

THE BURGER SPREADS

No, this chapter isn't about a particular show, but about some of the types of eating establishments that helped popularize the majestic burger.

DINERS

Diners are usually smallish restaurants with laid-back atmospheres, serving what can be best described as comfort food. Diners should have counter seating and booths where you can enjoy some music via tabletop jukeboxes while you wait for your food. I just described my ideal version of one, but yours might differ slightly. Typically, there's only one or two short-order cooks who handle all the cooking, an impressive thing to see up close. All good diners are open twenty-four-hours or at least into the wee hours of the night. I lump coffee shops into the same group as diners.

Many folks believe that the original diners were the lunch wagons of the late 1800s. Eventually, as the need for more seating arose, lunch wagons switched to prefabricated buildings. It wasn't until the 1960s and the advent of highways crisscrossing the United States that diners took off nationwide. Before this, most diners were found in small towns and urban areas.

DRIVE-INS

The drive-ins I'm referring to weren't the theater kind. At a drive-in restaurant, you would park your car and a member of their staff would come out to meet you at your vehicle, take your order, and then return with your food. Depending on the efficiency of the spot, you might have a quick meal or a drawn-out affair. Drive-ins rose to prominence as car culture took over America during the 1950s and 1960s; as folks got more comfortable using their cars for traveling from point A to point B, their "wheels" also started to become an extension of who they were.

Drive-ins are commonly associated with women skating around from hot rod to jalopy in the parking lot, but most, if not all, of the original carhops were guys or "tray boys." It wasn't until after World War II that women replaced men, after American males were called up to join the military. While it's true that having a pretty girl serve you food increased sales, in the long run it created problems with fellas loitering.

McDonald's found a way to streamline food service and cut out the problems with drive-in service. Once that new system spread to restaurants nationwide, the popularity of drive-ins began to wane. But it was the even more popular drive-thru service that would deal a major blow to drive-ins.

I wasn't around to experience the original drive-in. My first taste of it was watching Happy Days on TV. I dreamed of eating and hanging out at the Arnold's Drive-In featured on the program.

Believe it or not, there are actually a few hundred drive-ins still around where you can have your in-car eating experience. To find a list of all active drive-in restaurants with carhops, go to my blog, *Burger Beast*.

LUNCHEONETTES

Lunch counters or luncheonettes were initially just that, a counter where you could sit down on a stool to enjoy lunch. Waitresses would tend to the customers while a cook prepared the dish. Lunch counters were popularized inside five-and-dime stores, which had a twofold reason for being there. Hungry customers could stop and grab something to eat, and someone who had just dropped in for a bite might end up in the store buying something.

The menu kept it simple with things that could be cooked on a flat-top grill, like hamburgers, sandwiches, soups, and desserts. Breakfast was a favorite at most lunch counters. Specials like meatloaf or hot turkey could be found daily.

Lunch counters were hurt immensely by fast food fever in the United States. Unlike drive-ins, which have been able to carve out a living in smaller towns, lunch counters and luncheonettes have pretty much been wiped from existence.

DINERS, DRIVE-INS, AND LUNCH COUNTERS

A&W

Year Founded: *1919*
City Founded: *Lodi, California*
Founders: *Roy W. Allen & Frank Wright*
Number of Locations at the Chain's Peak: *over 2,300*
Slogan: *"All American Food"*

Roy W. Allen opened a small walk-up root beer stand in Lodi, California, on June 20, 1919. That night there was a party to celebrate the return of local World War I soldiers.

This was all happening the same year the Volstead Act was enacted. The prohibition of alcohol caused many to look for an alternative. Allen played on the phrase "root beer" to lure folks looking to get their alcoholic fill, even though root beer was no alcoholic beverage.

The success of the first stand led to the opening of a second one in Stockton, California, in the summer of 1920. Allen then partnered with his former employee Frank Wright. They leased the Lodi and Stockton locations and focused on an expansion into Sacramento, a much larger city.

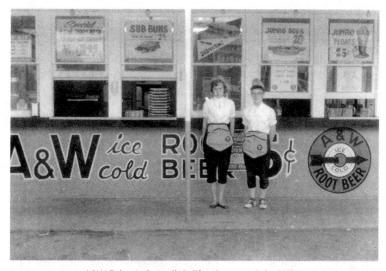

A&W Drive-In in Lodi, California around the 1920s.

Allen and Wright used the initials of their last names for their drink, "A&W Root Beer." Shortly afterward, a few more locations were opened in Houston, Texas.

In 1923, Allen decided to take advantage of the public's evolution into a more mobile society. He transformed one of the Sacramento root beer stands into a drive-in restaurant. The addition of "tray boys" to bring orders to thirsty customers changed the game. There are unsubstantiated claims that this was the first drive-in.

After buying out the company from Wright in 1924, Allen began to expand his brand by franchising across the United States the following year. He sold exclusive rights to the states of Arizona, California, Nevada, Oregon, and Washington to H.C. Bell and Lewis Reed. All of those locations would be renamed to "Reed & Bell Root Beer."

In 1927, J. Willard Marriott (yes, the hotel guy) bought the franchise rights for Baltimore, Maryland; Richmond, Virginia; and Washington, DC Later that year, he opened The Hot Shoppe, which would become the Hot Shoppes restaurant chain two years later.

A&W drive-ins continued to expand across the United States, and by 1933, there were over 170 of them. But after the US entered World War II, A&W Root Beer Drive-Ins suffered as much if not more than other restaurants of that era. Young men available to work the drive-ins were scarce. So were food, sugar, and other essentials to make the root beer. By the end of the war in 1945, nearly eighty A&W locations had closed up shop.

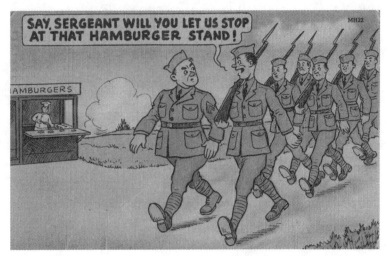

Hamburger Stand Postcard from 1942.

Once the franchise agreement for Reed and Bell expired in 1945, all the rights for those five states reverted to Allen. A boom for new franchisees saw over 450 A&W drive-ins in operation by 1950.

After Allen's wife took ill, he sold the company to a businessman named Gene Hurtz. During his tenure as owner, the drive-ins expanded their menus to have a more extensive selection of food. By 1963, the A&W brand had over 2,300 locations in the US, Canada, and Europe. In 1972, the Canadian restaurants were sold off separately and to this day operate independently of their US counterparts.

After a series of mergers and purchases, the company was owned by United Brands Company. A&W Root Beer Company became A&W International to reflect its growing global expansion. Part of their new marketing plan was to focus on the restaurants, not the root beer. In 1971, bottled A&W root beer was available in stores and markets across the US. Its popularity led to the formation of A&W Beverage, Inc. to sell root beer outside of the restaurants.

Drive-ins fell under the subsidiary of A&W Restaurants, Inc. as of 1978. United Brands sold off the restaurants in 1982 and followed that up the next year by selling off the beverage to a separate company. It was just like having two adopted brothers and sisters split up.

A&W Beverages ended up at Cadbury Schweppes in October, 1993, where it's now part of a soft drink portfolio that includes Crush, Dr. Pepper, RC Cola, and Seven-Up.

The restaurants are now franchisee-owned by A Great American Brand, LLC. Its headquarters are in Lexington, Kentucky, where they've got a new revamped A&W Burgers Chicken Floats concept that focuses on fresh beef burgers, hand-battered chicken tenders, and root beer that's made daily. I've visited one of the new stores and can't wait till they find their way to South Florida.

There are currently about 630 A&W restaurants in the US with another 370 in Southeast Asia. A&W in Canada is now privately owned and has over 850 locations.

Bob's Big Boy

Year Founded: *1936*
City Founded: *Glendale, California*
Founder: *Bob Wian*
Number of Locations at the Chain's Peak: *560*
Slogan: *"A Meal in One on a Double-Deck Bun"*

Big Boy founder Bob Wian started at the bottom. Shortly after graduating from high school in 1933, he took a job at the White Log Coffee Shop in

Los Angeles. He worked his way up from dishwasher to fry cook and then to manager. His boss at the time, Davis W. Wood, would later become the purchasing agent for the Bob's Big Boy chain. While at the White Log Coffee Shop, Wian learned their entire system of operation, from pricing to their use of a central commissary for all of their locations. Wian believed he could build a better mousetrap.

Wian was adamant about gaining restaurant experience, so he quit his management job and went back to an entry-level dishwashing gig at Rite Spot. He also learned the fry cook and counterman stations. The Rite Spot offered curb service, and Wian's younger sister was a carhop there. It was at Rite Spot that he learned how important consistency is in food service. The man who hired Wian at Rite Spot was Leonard A. Dunagan, who would later be the vice president and general manager of the Bob's Big Boy company. I guess it paid off to be kind to Wian.

Wian had been saving up his earnings to open up his own place. He came across a ten-stool stand located between a nursery and a liquor store in Glendale, California. He sold his DeSoto Roadster for three hundred dollars and used the proceeds to buy the store, then borrowed fifty dollars from his dad for supplies. On August 6, 1936, the stand reopened as Bob's Pantry.

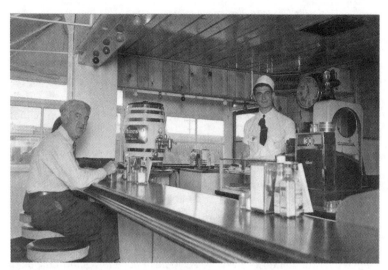

Bob Wian serving a customer at Bob's Pantry in 1936.

Bob's Big Boy Inspirations

Many of the dishes on the Bob's Pantry menu were "inspired" by dishes from his previous places of employment and restaurants that he frequented, like White Log's pancakes and C.C. Brown's Ice Cream Parlor's hot fudge sundae. The red hamburger relish from Rite Spot found its way onto the creation that would catapult Bob's Pantry into the world of burger legend.

In February 1937, members of the Glendale High School orchestra were having their usual burger meal when one of them asked for "something different, something special?" as he recalled in an interview for the *Milwaukee Journal* on December 16, 1958. It was that day that he created a sandwich that has been imitated a million times over, the original double-deck hamburger.

The original double-deck hamburger had a sesame bun that was sliced twice to create a middle piece of bread. If it sounds familiar, it's because it has had hundreds of restaurant imitators, including the most famous one, McDonald's Big Mac. I'm going to use McDonald's Big Mac lingo for the next paragraph: the bottom bun is the heel, the middle one is the club, and the sesame-seed top is the crown.

The heel was topped with a two-ounce beef patty, a slice of American cheese, and one and a half ounces of shredded lettuce with mayo, in that order. The club was placed on the bottom two-ounce beef patty. The upper half was stacked with red relish (sweet pickle relish, ketchup, and chili sauce), another two-ounce beef patty, and mayo, with the crown on top.

There are two different stories about the origins of the Big Boy burger name. One involves a chubby six-year-old named Richard Woodruff who helped out around Bob's Pantry. He was paid in burgers. A short time after the double-deck hamburger's creation, Wian called Woodruff "Big Boy," and the name stuck. There's also the rumor that Woodruff was originally nicknamed "Fat Boy," but the name couldn't be used because of a Fat Boy's Bar-B-Q restaurant, so they chose the next best thing, "Big Boy."

The original sketch for the iconic Big Boy character with the checkered overalls and burger in hand was drawn by Warner Brothers animation artist Ben Washam. Washam and Wian had worked together at the White Log Coffee Shop. Wian renamed Bob's Pantry after his now famous double-deck hamburger, Bob's Big Boy.

The Big Boy character would become as much of an icon as the sandwich. Large statues were erected outside restaurants and were famously stolen or kidnapped by pranksters. The Big Boy led to a favorite line of merchandising that exists to this day. I remember owning a Bob's Big Boy bank when I was a child.

Bob's Big Boy Licensing

Let's start calling Wian by his first name of Bob. It's a little friendlier. In 1938, a second Bob's Big Boy opened. The original location expanded, and curb service was added to both restaurants. Bob's sister Dottie moved over from Rite Spot to be a carhop at her brother's establishment.

It wasn't until the late 1940s that the Big Boy name would start to spread nationwide with the additions of Frisch's Big Boy (Cincinnati, Ohio), Eat'n Park Big Boy (Pittsburgh, Pennsylvania), Parkette Big Boy (Charleston, West Virginia; it became Shoney's Big Boy in 1954), and Elias Brothers Big Boy (Detroit, Michigan). Shoney's sub-franchised the Big Boy sandwich and name on behalf of Bob's Big Boy.

Bob was licensing to these franchisees the opportunity to sell his Big Boy double-deck hamburger, but not to use of the name of "Bob's Big Boy." This is why you normally found the words "Big Boy" proceeded with the possessive form of the owner's name.

How many exactly were there? Well, let's see. There was...

Abdow's, Arnold's, Azar's, Becker's, Bud's, Chez Chap, Don's, Eat'n Park, Elby's, Elias Brothers, Franklin's, Frejlach's, Frisch's, JB's (US), JB's (Canada), Kebo's, Ken's, Kip's, Lendy's, Leo's, Manners, Marc's, McDowell's, Mr. B's, Shap's, Shoney's, Ted's, TJ's, Tops, Tote's, Tune's, Vip's, and Yoda's.

I'm not even counting all of the chubby-kid imitator restaurants that sprouted up to try and catch some of that Bob's Big Boy magic.

Bob's Big Boy's Big Sales Meant Big Expansion

According to an ad in the *Van Nuys News* on November 7, 1951, the Bob's Big Boy had sold 2,600,000 Big Boy sandwiches with eight locations in operation.

In 1956, the original Bob's Big Boy location, or Bob's number one, as it was known, got a facelift and remodel. The newly designed and rebuilt drive-in, designed by architects Wayne McAllister and William C. Wagner, could now seat ninety customers inside along with fifty-five parking spaces outside for carhop service. The building was torn down in 1989 to make way for a mall.

On April 28, 1967, the twenty-three owned Bob's Big Boy restaurants and the five hundred or so franchised restaurants merged with Marriott-Hot Shoppes Inc. Yes, Marriott, the mammoth hotel chain—back then, they were primarily a food service company that also owned Hot Shoppes restaurants and seven hotels at the time of the merger. Marriott actually started as a root beer stand in 1927, but that's a story for another day.

Bob continued as president of the new "Big Boy Restaurants of America" division until his resignation in May 1968. Marriott began a rapid expansion of Bob's Big Boy that combined opening new locations with purchasing franchisees like JB's, Ken's, and Manners' stores.

Elias Brothers purchased the Big Boy trademark from Marriott in 1987. Marriott, however, kept the Bob's Big Boy name and the 208 Bob's Big Boy restaurants in operation. On December 18, 1989, Marriott announced that it was restructuring and focusing on its hotel brand. All of their Allie's (32 locations), Bickford's (31 locations), Bob's Big Boy (235 locations), Howard Johnson's (57 locations), Roy Rogers (358 locations), and Wag's (79 locations) restaurants would be sold.

In late January, 1991, 104 of the Marriott-owned Bob's Big Boys in California were sold with the plan for them to be converted to either Carrow's or Coco's restaurants. The rest of the Bob's Big Boy locations were sold off piecemeal over the next few years.

Bob's Big Boy Still Lives

In 2000, Robert Liggett purchased Big Boy Restaurants International from the bankrupt Elias Brothers. Shortly after that, Liggett made a deal with Frisch's Big Boy where he paid out $1.2 million for franchise rights in the states of Florida, Kansas, Oklahoma, and Texas. Frisch's would have the exclusive Big Boy rights in Indiana, Kentucky, and Ohio, excluding the Cleveland area.

The Bob's Big Boy location in Downey, California, is known as Bob's Big Boy Broiler, a drive-in restaurant with a Googie-style coffee shop. The building was originally erected in 1958. In its previous incarnation, it was known as Harvey's Broiler and later as Johnie's Broiler.

In 2002, the State of California's Historic Resources Commission registered the building as a Historic Landmark—which meant it was off limits for tearing it down. On Sunday, January 7, 2007, the current tenant of the property began to tear down the building without any permits. Police stopped the illegal demolition, and the fella responsible for it was later charged with five misdemeanor charges for his trouble.

Out of this debacle, one hero rose from the ashes. Jim Louder, owner of the Bob's Big Boy in Torrance, signed a ninety-nine-year lease with the property owner with help from the Downey Historical Society, and Downey's Redevelopment Agency rebuilt it. Whatever parts of the structure survived from the demolition were incorporated into the new restaurant. The original blueprints were used to keep it as authentic as possible.

Denny's

> Year Founded: *1953*
> City Founded: *Lakewood, California*
> Founders: *Harold Butler & Richard Jezak*
> Number of Locations: *currently over 1,700*
> Slogan: *"America's diner is always open."*

In 1953, Harold Butler and Richard Jezak opened a nine-hundred-square-foot donut shop in Lakewood, California, called Danny's Do-Nuts, selling donuts filled with jam (not jelly) and high-grade coffee. Instantly successful, they quickly added a second location in Garden Grove that was twice the size. It was not as well received, so they added a grill to sell hamburgers.

Jezak left the company in 1955, and a year later Butler changed to a twenty-four-hour coffee shop with the opening of the eighth restaurant. Danny's Do-Nuts would now be known as Danny's Coffee Shops "to serve the best cup of coffee, make the best donuts, give the best service, offer the best value, and stay open twenty-four hours a day."

In 1959, Butler worried that customers might confuse Danny's Coffee Shops with the Los Angeles restaurant chain Coffee Dan's. So the name was changed to Denny's Coffee Shops and then shortened to Denny's in 1961.

Butler saw the car revolution in California and had the foresight to build a restaurant chain to fill those needs. He is considered by many to have pioneered fast service, high volume, low prices, and menus that were uniform at every location. Franchising started in 1963, and by 1981 there were well over a thousand restaurants. Denny's even converted a bunch of former Sambo's restaurant locations and made minimal changes to the building and sign design.

A Denny's Classic Diner concept opened in Fort Myers on May 13, 1997. The three thousand-square-foot prefabricated building emulates a 1950s diner. The Denny's Classic Diner, which seats 117 customers, has since added more locations in the United States. It's funny to see things come full circle like this.

Denny's Quirky Facts

In 1977, the Grand Slam breakfast was introduced at an Atlanta Denny's location. It was a nod to baseball player Hank Aaron, who three years earlier had bested Babe Ruth's home run record.

Denny's famously attempted to close for the first time on Christmas Day 1988. The only problem was that seven hundred locations had either lost their keys or never even had locks. All but about fifty to sixty franchised locations stayed open for the holiday.

Dog 'n Suds

Year Founded: *1953*
City Founded: *Champaign, Illinois*
Founders: *James Griggs & Don Hamacher*
Number of Locations at the Chain's Peak: *650*
Slogan: *"...Where Everything's So Dog-gone Good!"*

Champaign High School orchestra director Jim Griggs and chorus director Don Hamacher had heard about a coach in a neighboring town who was running a successful root beer stand. They figured they too could make a go of it.

Griggs reached out to an acquaintance, a graduate student at a nearby university, who created the layout and design of the restaurant. He then constructed a model of his drive-in creation and called it Dog 'n Suds. Why that name? The student said the name embraced what they were selling: hot dogs and suds, a slang word for root beer. The name stuck.

Griggs, who was giving violin lessons to the children of attorney John Franklin, told him about the idea for Dog 'n Suds and his business plan. Franklin not only helped find their first location but financed the project and gave them legal advice.

In 1953, Dog 'n Suds opened in Champaign, Illinois, as a drive-in, employing Hamacher's and Griggs' students as carhops. On the first day, with only Coney dogs and root beer on the menu, they did three hundred dollars in sales. Hamacher's wife Maggie created the Coney sauce for the hot dogs and Reed and Bell was the brand of root beer they served.

So many cars lined up at the Dog 'n Suds the first week that police officers showed up to direct traffic at night. The success of Dog 'n Suds led Hamacher and Griggs to leave behind their life of education and embrace their newfound profession, which was multiplying quickly via franchising.

What made being a franchisee of Dog 'n Suds so attractive was that there was only a one-time franchise fee and no royalty percentage to be paid to the corporation. The first franchise was sold to a woman who inquired about franchising just a week after opening. Her Dog 'n Suds opened shortly afterward in Rantoul, Illinois. Before they knew it, Dog 'n Suds drive-ins sprouted up all over Illinois. In quick succession, the states of Indiana, Ohio, and Michigan followed.

By 1960, the famous Dog 'n Suds "World's Creamiest Root Beer" recipe and equipment had been developed. *Forbes* rated Dog 'n Suds as one of the top-growing franchises in the 1960s. There was even a training center in Champaign named Rover College after their mascot. The eight-day course covered the technical, marketing and administrative aspects of the Dog 'n Suds business. Upon graduation, grads would receive a master of drive-inology degree.

At their peak in 1968, there were over six hundred Dog 'n Suds locations in thirty-eight states and Canada, with approximately fifteen new restaurants opening each month.

In 1969, Franklin, who was in poor health, together with Griggs, wanted to sell their shares of the company. Hamacher got four of his friends to buy out Franklin and Griggs. At this point, many of their food contemporaries had gone public, and Hamacher thought that Dog 'n Suds could too. Unfortunately, the Minnie Pearl debacle which also derailed Royal Castle killed those chances. Dog 'n Suds was sold to American Licensing Company in 1970.

By the time that Dog 'n Suds moved their HQ to Arlington Heights, Illinois, in 1972, the number of Dog 'n Suds locations was hovering around 450. Rover College had also found a new home in Arlington.

Dog 'n Suds agreed to merge with Frostie Enterprises; they not only sold their own branded root beer but also owned 120 Stewart's Drive-In locations. On August 12, 1975, Frostie bought out the majority stake in Dog 'n Suds for $750,000. Frostie implemented cost cutting measures that hurt Dog 'n Suds on the franchise front. They also made the crazy decision to change their root beer recipe, which did not sit well with longtime fans.

Many Dog 'n Suds locations either dropped the name and rebranded or closed altogether. No new restaurants were opening at this point, and by the end of 1975, they were down to 350 drive-ins. The newfound popularity of drive-thrus didn't help things either. By 1978, the Dog 'n Suds company had shrunk to 140 restaurants. The following year, the retail root beer business and restaurants were sold to two separate companies.

There were only twenty-four Dog 'n Suds left in 1990 when the company was sold again. Just when things seemed hopeless, a shining light appeared out of the darkness. Don Van Dame, whose father had opened the first Indiana franchise of Dog 'n Suds, his wife Carol, and his partner, Dick Morath, purchased the Dog 'n Suds trademark in 1991. That same year they started selling the "World's Creamiest Root Beer" to supermarkets in the Midwest. In 2001, they created a new company to license the Dog 'n Suds brand. The Van Dames entered into an exclusive agreement with Clover Club Bottling Co. in 2006 to have them bottle their root beer.

Currently, there are fourteen Dog 'n Suds locations where you can still get your Coney dogs, Root Beer, and Char-Co Burgers. If you're in the Muskegon, Michigan, area, hit up my friend David Hosticka's Dog 'n Suds and check out all the great historical pieces on display.

Howard Johnson's

Year Founded: *1925*
City Founded: *Quincy, Massachusetts*
Founder: *Howard Deering Johnson*
Number of Locations at the Chain's Peak: *over 1,000*
Slogan: *"Landmark for Hungry Americans"*

With five hundred dollars borrowed from his recently widowed mother and another two thousand dollars from family friend Dr. George Dalton, Howard Deering Johnson bought the Walker-Barlow drugstore on Beale Street in the Wollaston neighborhood of Quincy, Massachusetts, where he had been working. The newly revamped Howard Johnson's opened its doors on September 23, 1925; it featured a marble soda fountain and sold candies, cigars, magazines, newspapers, sodas and three flavors of ice cream (chocolate, strawberry, and vanilla).

Johnson decided to tinker with the ice cream being served. He doubled the butterfat, and that would ultimately be a game changer for him. Another important factor was the all-natural ingredients used, nothing artificial.

The popularity of the ice cream allowed him to open a twenty-two-foot stand attached to a house on Wollaston Beach in the summer of 1926. On the first Sunday, the new spot took in two hundred dollars. By the end of the summer, it was so busy that on one Sunday in particular, fourteen thousand cones were sold. Over those few months, the new location generated more revenue than the Beale Street location had earned since opening. The following summer, hot dogs and soft drinks were added, along with two new stands at Nantasket Beach in Hull and at Revere Beach.

In June, 1929, Johnson opened his first restaurant in the only high-rise in the city at the time, Quincy Square's Granite Trust. The restaurant featured traditional New England foods and his now famous twenty-eight flavors of ice cream. Its location at a busy intersection made it an instant success.

John Eagles Alcott was responsible for the memorable "Simple Simon and the Pieman" logo, based on an old English nursery rhyme. He was also responsible for the orange-and-teal color scheme and font used in the Howard Johnson's logo.

In 1929, the beginning of the Great Depression caused him to begin franchising the Howard Johnson's concept. All of the franchisees would purchase all of the food and supplies from a commissary and be allowed to use the Howard Johnson's name, the iconic orange tiles, and the logo that was so closely associated with the brand. During this time, many others emulated his vision for franchising.

As more Americans bought cars and took to the roads for travel, new highways and byways sprouted up. Johnson chose interstate highways and major intersections as locations for the new restaurants. Known as a "Landmark for Hungry Americans," Howard Johnson's could be found across the United States. By 1936, there were sixty-one total "Howard Johnson's," forty-eight ice cream shops and restaurants, and thirteen roadside and beach stands.

When you entered a Howard Johnson's restaurant, you'd find a counter with stools where you could take a load off and grab your favorite ice cream or a hot dog. Looking for something more formal? In the dining room, you could enjoy a full meal.

Their famous ice cream was made with milk and cream from the H.P. Hood Company in Charleston, Massachusetts. Below are the twenty-eight flavors, in order of popularity. I'd have thought Butter Pecan would have done better.

► Vanilla	► Banana	► Orange-Pineapple
► Chocolate	► Peach	► Pecan Brittle
► Chocolate Chip	► Peppermint	► Butterscotch
► Strawberry	► Burgundy Cherry	► Black Raspberry
► Coffee	► Butter Pecan	► Pineapple
► Maple Walnut	► Caramel Fudge	► Fruit Salad
► Pistachio	► Frozen Pudding	► Coconut
► Butter Crunch	► Macaroon	► Lemon

- ▸ Grape Nut
- ▸ Peanut Brittle
- ▸ Ginger
- ▸ Apple

There were orange, raspberry, lime, and lemon sherbet flavors on the menu, too.

During World War II, Howard Johnson's tried to sustain itself by selling food to government workers. The number of locations dwindled from two hundred to just about a dozen. A few years after the war was over, they began construction on two hundred new restaurants throughout the South and Midwest. By 1954, there were nearly four hundred locations in thirty-two states. In this rebound year, they opened the first Howard Johnson's motor lodge in Savannah, Georgia.

By the time Howard Brennan Johnson took the reins from his retired dad in 1959, Howard Johnson's had 675 restaurants and 175 motor lodges. The number of company locations took a little dip when they went public in 1961, but still included 605 restaurants, eighty-eight motor lodges, and ten Red Coach Grill restaurants, a chain they had purchased in the early 1960s.

Chefs Pierre Franey and Jacques Pépin were hired by Howard Brennan Johnson to supervise and develop recipes at the main Howard Johnson's commissary in Brockton, Massachusetts. The signature dishes were flash-frozen to ensure a consistent product when it was delivered across the country.

Howard Johnson's would peak a few years later with almost one thousand restaurants and 550 motor lodge in forty-two states, the District of Columbia, the Bahamas, the British West Indies, Canada, and Puerto Rico. There was also a supermarket line of branded Howard Johnson's frozen foods, soft drinks, and ice cream.

In 1979, the Imperial Group Limited bought the Howard Johnson's empire for $630 million, then sold it to the Marriott Corporation in 1985 for $314 million. Marriott converted the four hundred-plus company owned HoJo locations to Bob's Big Boy restaurants. It seems Marriott was more interested in the real estate on which the restaurants sat than anything else.

The dejected Howard Johnson restaurant franchisees were fearful that they might be put out of business. In 1986, they incorporated as the Franchise Associates. Marriott gave them the rights to operate and maintain Howard Johnson's restaurants. Forty-four of them located in twenty-six states continued to use the Howard Johnson name. By the time Franchise Associates ceased operations in 2005, there were only a handful of restaurants still open. As of this writing, there is one last standing Howard Johnson's restaurant in Lake George, New York, which is only a Howard Johnson's in name; it no longer has any of their signature dishes or ice cream.

I did not mention hamburgers even once in this historical recap, but I have fond memories of eating hamburgers at Howard Johnson's when I was a little boy during our family's yearly road trips. Burgers were a popular dish for weary travelers, and all those locations scattered across the US helped spread the popularity of the hamburger.

SONIC

> Year Founded: *1953*
> City Founded: *Shawnee, Oklahoma*
> Founder: *Troy Smith*
> Number of Locations at the Chain's Peak: *currently over 3,600*
> Slogan: *"This Is How You SONIC"*

In 1953, Troy Smith purchased a parcel of land in Shawnee, Oklahoma, that had a log house and a walk-up root beer stand by the name of Top Hat. During a trip to Louisiana in 1954, after visiting a drive-in where orders were placed via speakers, he had an epiphany.

Smith converted the stand into a drive-in by adding parking spaces, canopies, carhops, and an intercom system for ordering. Sales tripled. Record numbers of hamburgers with tiny top hat toothpicks sticking out of them were delivered by carhops.

Smith partnered with Charlie Pappe in 1956 to open a second Top Hat Drive-In in Woodward, Oklahoma. In 1958, after having opened additional Top Hat Drive-in locations in Enid and Stillwater, they tried to copyright the name. It was already taken.

Inspired by America's obsession with everything related to space and the atomic age, they went with the name SONIC. The short name also worked in their favor since they wanted to add a neon sign, which could get expensive. SONIC matched up perfectly with the Top Hat slogan, "Service with the Speed of Sound."

Pappe and Smith sat down with a lawyer to come up with a straightforward franchise agreement. Initially, they would make a penny off of each SONIC-label hamburger bag sold, which they would split. It wasn't until later that any marketing or standardized operations would be put into effect company-wide.

A supply and distribution division named SONIC Supply was created to help the growing company in the 1960s. By the time Pappe passed away in 1967, there were forty-one SONIC drive-ins; five years later, the chain was regional, with about 165 locations in Arkansas, Kansas, Oklahoma, and Texas by 1972.

In 1973, SONIC Supply was restructured as a franchise company to provide franchisees with needed equipment and any necessary instructions for running a SONIC. Five years later, they opened their one thousandth drive-in in Midwest City, Oklahoma.

By the time the 1980s rolled around, SONIC was operating more like a group of loosely associated independent restaurants than a chain. And even though Smith had retired in 1983, he still enjoyed attending the grand opening celebrations for new SONIC restaurants.

Under J. Clifford Hudson's leadership, first as president in 1995 and then as CEO of SONIC (his current status as of 2000), the company refocused their efforts to create the unified operational and marketing vision for the company that is in place now. There are now over 3,600 SONIC restaurants located in forty-five states.

SONIC Beach?

SONIC Beach, a new beach-themed concept that serves beer and wine, opened up in Homestead, Florida, in June of 2011. In November of that same year, the location at Fort Lauderdale Beach took the SONIC beach idea to the next level. It features an outdoor seating area that overlooks the beach and the Atlantic Ocean. A few other SONIC beach locations have opened since in South Florida.

Woolworth

> Year Founded: *1879*
> City Founded: *Utica, New York*
> Founder: *Frank Winfield Woolworth*
> Number of Locations at the Chain's Peak: *over 3,000*
> Slogan: *"Woolworth's Great Five Cent Store"*

Today's younger generation has no idea about Woolworth's mega-popularity back in the day. It could best be compared to the juggernaut that Walmart or Amazon is now.

Woolworth is probably best remembered as a five-and-dime, a store that sold inexpensive personal and household items. Frank Winfield Woolworth's first store location opened in Utica, New York, on February 22, 1879. The thirteen by twenty feet store made fifty dollars on its first day in operation. By June 1879, it was out of business.

But on June 21, 1879, he struck gold with his second location in Lancaster, Pennsylvania. This slightly larger store (fourteen by twenty-five feet) sold $128 on its first day, enough to prove that the concept had legs.

On August 31, 1910, the first official Woolworth eatery opened its doors on 14th Street in New York City. The Refreshment Room, as it was known, came from a phrase that Woolworth had heard in England. Unlike the Formica counters that Woolworth's would be remembered for, this restaurant featured fancier glass-topped marble tables. The Refreshment

Room (twenty-seven by sixty feet) was found at the back of Woolworth. The walls were full of artwork, and the smell of fresh flowers filled the room. Uniformed waiters and waitresses served food on fine china and made sure that all customers had a pleasant experience.

After the success of this location, Frank opened a second one in Lancaster at the new store in the Woolworth Skyscraper. Of the over 37,000 folks who showed up on opening day, 3,279 sampled a free tasting meal. Fried oysters were the favorite dish, and nothing on the menu cost more than ten cents. By the time 1928 rolled around, Woolworth was serving ninety million meals per day.

After World War II, Woolworth's Refreshment Rooms were replaced with the luncheonettes with their memorable Formica counters. The company also introduced special in-house food promotions like the popular Roast Turkey Dinner.

The Woolworth eateries included bakeries, cafeterias, sit-down and stand-up counters, and soda fountains. The lines for breakfast and lunch at the luncheonettes were long because they were one of the few reasonably priced quick-service eateries. Keeping all of their customers well fed with grilled cheese sandwiches and hamburgers made Woolworth one of the largest food purveyors in the world.

An essential part of the Woolworth Luncheonette experience was the Woolworth's waitress. They usually wore aprons, caps, and a Woolworth-issued uniform. Depending on the size of the eatery, she may have also been the cook.

If you love sitting at the counter where all the action happens as I do, then you know there's usually some lingo that exists between waitresses and the short-order cook who makes your greasy spoon goodness. It was no different at Woolworth. According to DinerLingo.com, these are some of the phrases we burgers fans might hear:

BESSIE!	Roast Beef or Hamburger
BLACK WATER!	Root Beer
BURGER WITH BREATH!	Hamburger with onions
BURN ONE!	Put a hamburger on the grill
BUTCHER'S REVENGE!	Meatloaf
DRAG ONE THROUGH WISCONSIN!	Put cheese on it
HOCKEY PUCK!	Well-done hamburger
SIDE OF JOAN OF ARC!	French fries
TWO COWS, MAKE 'EM CRY!	Two hamburgers with onions
YELLOW BLANKET ON A DEAD COW!	Cheeseburger

During the 1960s, Woolworth introduced Harvest House restaurants in shopping malls and Red Grilles in their Woolco stores. At the time, eighty percent of Woolworth locations had some sort of eatery located inside.

The late 1960s and 1970s brought in a wave of fast-food restaurants that began to dominate and change the eating landscape of the United States. There were still hundreds of the "outdated" lunch counters like the ones found at Woolworth and their contemporaries that had not changed one bit in over fifty years. They began to suffer financially.

As the number of Woolworth stores began winding down in the late 1990s, so did all of the eateries. All of those who worked the lunch counters were the first to go, and every last piece of equipment, from coffee mugs to ice cream dishes, was sold off. Many folks never even got a chance to say goodbye and have one last cheeseburger or ice cream float before the end. It is sad that such an iconic part of American food culture disappeared so quickly.

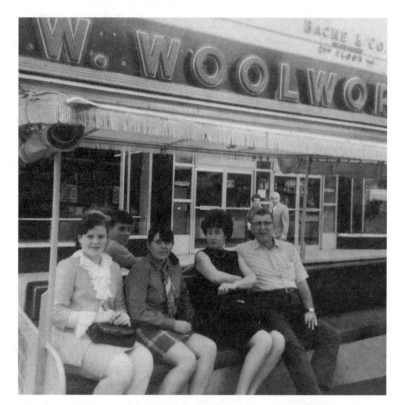

Burger Beast's mom Cary, uncle Francisco, aunt Rosa and grandparents Juana & Gregorio outside of a Woolworth in 1964 New York.

If you ever find yourself in Bakersfield, California, then seek out the Five & Dime Antique Mall, where a fully functioning former Woolworth Luncheonette is located in the back corner of the building. The Woolworth Diner has counter seats, Formica tables, a lunch counter, and best of all, food. The open kitchen will bring you back to a simpler time. Order a yellow blanket on a dead cow with a side of Joan of Arc and some black water to wash it all down.

Chapter

4

MCDONALD'S

McDonald's is the best-known burger joint in the world. There's no disputing that fact when they've got more than 35,000 locations in over 120 countries. McDonald's story is interesting. If you watched the movie *The Founder* starring Michael Keaton, you may think you already know it. The filmmakers used creative license to tell the story of McDonald's, however, so it wasn't exactly like that.

BOREDOM LEADS TO CREATIVITY

Originally from Manchester, New Hampshire, Maurice (Mac) and Richard (Dick) McDonald moved to California in the summer of 1928 searching for fame, fortune, or a little of both in the growing film industry.

Both Mac and Dick found jobs as stagehands working on movie sets for Columbia Movie Studios, not precisely what they had envisioned. By 1930, they were able to save enough money to purchase a 750-seat vaudeville theater near Glendale, California, which they renamed the Beacon. It didn't bring them the monetary windfall they were hoping for. They were only really making money at the concession stand.

HELLO BBQ, GOODBYE BBQ

After selling the theater in 1937, they decide to switch gears and open "The Airdrome" in Monrovia, California, an octagon-shaped open-air hot dog stand that featured fresh squeezed orange juice. They moved their shack to San Bernardino, California, and renamed the newly redesigned and expanded building McDonald's Barbecue (spelled Bar-B-Q on the sign outside) on May 15, 1940.

McDonald's Barbecue was a drive-in with no indoor seating. It did, however, have carhops, along with a barbecue heavy menu with twenty-five items, one of which was the mighty hamburger. The restaurant was a success, but the brothers were growing, well, indifferent.

"We just became bored," Dick recalled in an interview before his passing. "The money was coming in, and there wasn't much for us to do."

New Systems Come Into Place

In October 1948, they closed for three months to revamp their booming business. During this time, they erected a giant sign informing everyone they were closed for alterations and that America's first 'Drive-in Hamburger Bar' would be opening soon.

On December 20, 1948, the McDonald brothers unleashed a new type of restaurant, just "McDonald's." Gone were the jukebox, vending machines, telephones, and anything that would encourage teenagers to loiter. The menu was scaled down to just hamburgers, cheeseburgers, milk, coffee, three different soft drinks, potato chips, and pie. The potato chips and pie didn't make the cut and were later replaced by milkshakes and french fries.

While these changes might seem significant, the most important alteration they made was to introduce the "McDonald's New Self-Service System" featuring fifteen-cent hamburgers. The carhops were gone. Now, customers were expected to walk up to one of the two service windows and place an order. They had to eat in their car or take the food home, because other than a few benches, there was not much in the way of seating. Paper wrappers and cups replaced all the dinnerware and silverware. You even had to get rid of your own trash.

The kitchen was set up like an assembly line where everyone in the twelve-person crew had a specialized job, like manning the grill or adding the condiments. The standardization meant all hamburgers (ten to a pound) were topped with ketchup, mustard, onions, and two pickles, unless requested otherwise.

One of the more exciting creations that came out of the new system was the automatic condiment dispenser. This would squirt an exact amount of ketchup or mustard at the press of a button. Another innovation was the use of infrared lamps to keep the food warm.

It was all about efficiency and saving money wherever they could on the daily operation of the business, because they didn't make much money per food item. The operation only became lucrative when everything was sold in larger quantities.

I'm sure the McDonald brothers expected there to be a learning curve to this new way of doing business. But initially, the new McDonald's did not click with customers. Customers got angry waiting for carhops who never showed or didn't like having to pay beforehand for their meal.

But after four months, the tide had turned, and people from all walks of life, and in particular, families wanted to eat at McDonald's. They weren't the only ones. Folks with ambitions to own or upgrade their burger restaurants began to show up. The brothers took it in stride and shared their secrets with the interested parties. One visitor of note who was given the full tour by the McDonald brothers in 1952 was Keith Cramer, who went on to cofound Insta Burger King in Jacksonville, Florida, the following year. Insta Burger King would later become Burger King, but we'll get into that in the next chapter.

The brothers begin franchising in 1952 with Neil Fox from Phoenix, Arizona, plunking down a franchise fee of one thousand dollars. He insisted on using the McDonald's name, which was not part of the deal and wasn't even known outside of San Bernardino.

It was the first location to use the golden arches design with the red and white tiles for which McDonald's later became known. The twenty-five-foot arches were Dick McDonald's idea, brought to life by architect Stanley Clark Meston. Dick wanted something to catch the eye of passing motorists. McDonald's first mascot SpeeDee made his debut on an animated neon sign at another smaller arch by the street. SpeeDee, a cartoonish small man with a hamburger-shaped face, wore a chef's jacket and striped pants. He was winking out of one eye and appeared to be walking fast.

Fox's second McDonald's location in Phoenix opened in May 1953. A few months later, his brother-in-law Roger Williams and his business partner Burdette Landon opened the third location in Downey, California.

The first two McDonald's buildings are no longer around, making the Downey location the oldest restaurant in the chain still in operation. It looks pretty much as it did in 1953, because the franchise agreement was with the McDonald brothers and not with the later McDonald's Corporation, so they were not required to update their look.

ENTER RAY KROC

To keep up with demand for their famous milkshakes, Dick and Mac purchased eight of the five spindle Multimixers made by Prince Castle. Each spindle allowed five shakes per machine to be made at one time. Prince Castle Multimixers were sold by Ray Kroc, whose interest was piqued when an order came in for eight of them. Back then, even the busiest ice cream parlor would make do with just one of these machines.

Ray became so enamored with McDonald's that he offered to help them franchise the brand throughout the country. William Tansey was already selling franchises for the brothers, but he had just suffered a heart attack and was at home convalescing. This opened the door for Ray to work his magic.

Ray returned to his home in a Chicago suburb with the rights to franchise McDonald's throughout the US, except for the few spots that the brothers had already licensed in California and Arizona. The deal in place was rather simple: Dick and Mac were to receive one-half of one percent of the new franchises' gross sales.

On March 2, 1955, Ray Kroc founded McDonald's Systems, Inc. through which to sell his franchises. The following month, he opened his own McDonald's in Des Plaines, Illinois. The sales for the first day were $366.12, the equivalent of about $3,400 today.

Eugene Wright of Wright's Decorating Service came up with an interior color scheme for the Des Plaines location: yellow and white with dark brown and red as secondary trim colors. The exterior featured, of course, the golden arches design.

Ray hired Fred L. Turner as a grill man after Fred was unable to secure financing to open his own McDonald's. Fred would later become a significant figure in company history as CEO and Chairman. His attention to detail was essential since they were continually trying to improve the system created by the McDonald brothers. Without a doubt, Fred was Ray Kroc's right hand during those initial years.

Now that his McDonald's in Des Plaines was open, Ray could focus on finding franchisees. By 1958, McDonald's had sold its one hundred millionth hamburger, and it passed the hundred-restaurant location mark in Fond du Lac, Wisconsin, the following year.

CHANGING THE WAY THEY DO BUSINESS

Harry Sonneborn, who worked for the Tastee Freez ice cream and restaurant chain, approached Ray Kroc with an innovative way to deal with franchises. Kroc's company would borrow from institutions and operate as more of a real estate company, since a hamburger company would have much more difficulty getting funding.

The new McDonald's Franchise Realty Corporation would buy land in carefully selected locations, then turn around and rent the space to McDonald's franchisees. It allowed them to keep control of franchise operations. If the franchise owner decided to violate any part of the agreement, McDonald's could evict them.

Ray Kroc's company was rechristened the McDonald's Corporation in 1960. That same year, the "Look for the Golden Arches" advertising campaign was a big success for them.

The year 1961 was game-changing for McDonald's. Ray Kroc was growing increasingly frustrated with the McDonald brothers, particularly when it came to decisions that needed to be made affecting the entire company. Ray decided to ask them point-blank what would it cost for them to sell the company to him. The brothers wanted $2.7 million, which would net each of them a million after taxes. Ray came up with the funds from a variety of investors, including Princeton University.

The brothers did make one mistake, though. While they still owned the original McDonald's location, they were forced to rename it because they were no longer affiliated with the McDonald's Corporation. The original location, renamed "The Big M," was left to some of their loyal employees—for them not only to run but own it. It had a pretty good nine-year run. Later, Kroc opened a McDonald's just one block north.

Fred Turner's Hamburger University at the McDonald's in Elk Grove Village, Illinois, also opened in 1961. Each employee trainee originally got thirty-two hours of training. Hamburger University's future managers learned to develop their skills in categories such as leadership, operations, business growth, and customer appreciation. The original "classroom" was located in the basement of the restaurant. The first graduating class of fifteen received a "Bachelor of Hamburgerology" degree.

As of 2018, more than eighty thousand people have graduated from Hamburger University. Campuses are now located in Oak Brook, Illinois, US; Sydney, Australia; Munich, Germany; London, England; Tokyo, Japan; São Paulo, Brazil; and Shanghai, China.

In the early 1960s, McDonald's used market research to find out what customers identified with. The new golden arches logo bested the SpeeDee character in 1962. Meanwhile, the first McDonald's location with seating opened in Denver, Colorado.

The following year, Willard Scott, who played Bozo the Clown in the Washington, DC, market, was tapped to be Ronald McDonald. This scary Ronald looked nothing like the one popularized a few years later in all the McDonaldland ads and commercials.

ONE BILLION HAMBURGERS SOLD

By 1963, McDonald's hit the one billion hamburgers sold mark in their five hundred locations. When the company finally went public in 1965, its common shares were offered at $22.50 per share. If you had bought one hundred shares back in the day, it would be valued at almost ten million dollars today. In 1980, the McDonald's Corporation became one of the companies that make up the Dow Jones Industrial Average.

In 1968, McDonald's signature burger, the Big Mac, was rolled out nationwide to all restaurants. Originally known as the Aristocrat and the Blue Ribbon burger, the Big Mac had been created a year earlier by Jim Delligatti, a McDonald's franchisee in Pittsburgh, Pennsylvania. The Big Mac was his answer to Eat'n Park's Big Boy Sandwich, the original double-deck hamburger.

The style of the brown mansard roof locations with indoor seating was perhaps spurred on by Burger King's redesign and addition of indoor seating in 1967. The first such McDonald's made its debut in 1969 in Matteson, Illinois. At the same time, McDonald's had finally opened at least one restaurant in each state.

MCDONALDLAND

Advertising agency Needham Harper & Steers are credited with creating the McDonaldland characters (Ronald McDonald, the Hamburglar, Mayor McCheese, Officer Big Mac, Grimace, Captain Crook, Mad Professor, and Goblins, later known as Fry Guys) in 1971.

Then Don Ament and his company Setmakers were hired to bring them to life for TV commercials. McDonald's liked the original set he built so much that they decided to have themed playgrounds at some locations.

The very first McDonaldland Playland opened in Chula Vista, California, in 1971. The playground featured wall decor, swings, teeter-totters, and statues with Ronald McDonald and friends.

Sierra Vista, Arizona, has the distinction of being the first McDonald's restaurant with a drive-thru. It opened in 1975 when the goal of the company was to take care of the customer in fifty seconds or less. Of course, this was before McDonald's had expanded their menu. Today, the drive-thru accounts for about 70 percent of their total sales.

In 1979, the company launched the McDonald's Happy Meal: a hamburger or cheeseburger, french fries, cookies, a soft drink, and a toy. It had a circus wagon theme.

MCDLT

Ray Kroc passed away on January 14, 1984, at the age of eighty-one. It was the same year that McDonald's debuted the McDLT, its most infamous sandwich. The McDLT came in a specially designed container where the left side kept the top bun, cheese, lettuce, and tomato cool while the bottom bun and hamburger patty were on the hot side. You would open the container and put your burger together. The McDLT will live on in everyone's memory for two reasons: the Styrofoam container the burger was housed in, and the so-bad-it's-good commercial featuring Jason Alexander of Seinfeld fame.

How has McDonald's been able to survive when many of its contemporaries have either gone out business or been bought and merged with other chains?

McDonald's has an uncanny knack for reinventing itself and getting ahead of trends before it's too late. The last ten years have seen a better burger movement in the US, where fresh never-frozen patties are important to the consumer. The last time McDonald's sold fresh beef patties was the early 1970s. But in early 2018, they announced that they were switching all of their quarter-pound burgers to fresh beef, cooked to order. It's only a matter of time before the smaller patties follow suit. I only ask one thing, don't mess with the fries, speaking of which...

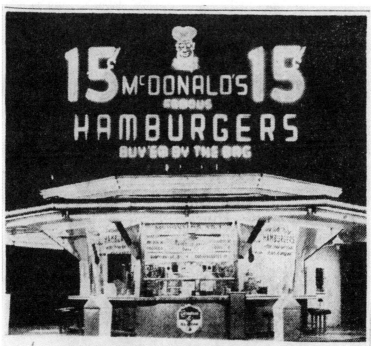

McDonald's ad announcing the addition of french fries from the *San Bernardino County Sun* on March 25, 1950.

MCDONALD'S FRIES

French fries have been high on the McDonald's priority list for the last seventy years. It goes all the way back to Mac McDonald, who devoted countless hours to perfecting their french fry recipe. Back then, the fries were fresh cut and made with Idaho russets.

Interstate Foods, the company who supplied McDonald's shortening, was too small to afford the equipment necessary to create the partially hydrogenated oil everyone was using for frying foods. Interstate Foods founder Harry Smargon came up with an alternative: a blend of 7 percent vegetable oil and 93 percent beef tallow (fat). This particular shortening blend created the crispy on the outside, soft on the inside, flavorful fry that became associated with McDonald's.

Once Ray Kroc got involved, he realized fries were critically important to what made McDonald's special. Plenty of restaurants had great burgers. But how many had an incredible french fry?

Potatoes vary in their water content, which can create soggy fries, so consistency was important. Kroc sent out field men with hydrometers to make sure that all of McDonald's potato suppliers were producing potatoes with the ideal solids amount of twenty to twenty-three percent.

In order to get crispy fries, sugars in potatoes need to be converted to starch. Kroc would cure the potatoes by storing them under a giant fan in the basement of his first restaurant. This french fry ritual was crucial in producing the perfect spud.

After hiring electrical engineer Louis Martino to create a "potato computer," cooking times for fries became standardized so that every McDonald's restaurant would deliver the perfect fry.

In 1966, Ray Kroc began phase out fresh cut fries, but that was OK as long as their secret weapon did not change. Formula 47, the unique cooking oil blend, was named after McDonald's "All American Meal," which included a fifteen-cent burger, a twelve-cent order of fries, and a twenty-cent milkshake.

Along Ray Kroc's journey of perfecting the art of making the french fry, he met J.R. Simplot from Boise, Idaho. Not only was Simplot the largest producer of frozen potatoes in the US, he had also cultivated a technique for growing the ideal Idaho russet potato year-round. After a handshake agreement with Kroc, Simplot agreed to build a factory to produce McDonald's fries.

McDonald's was the gold standard for french fries until the 1980s' health kick hit. On July 23, 1990, they caved in to the public pressure over the amount of saturated fat in their fries. They changed both their fry recipe and their frying oil to a blend of vegetable oils. While supposedly healthier with less cholesterol and saturated fat, the new oil blend had one major thing going against it: the fries were no longer as tasty as they once were. And the new oil was high in trans fat, which is even worse than saturated fat.

Since then, McDonald's has tinkered with their fries, but they've never returned to the flavor they had in the pre-1990 glory years. One last note: the current version of McDonald's fries is not vegan- or vegetarian-friendly, which means we can still hold out hope for an original beef tallow french fry revival.

MCDONALD'S DUNK CUP

Having ketchup with your french fries is as commonplace as cheese on a hamburger. But it wasn't always that way. McDonald's fries were never really meant to be eaten any other way than alone. All of the ketchup at McDonald's was used exclusively to top the burgers.

Then customers started asking for ketchup to enjoy with their fries. The company policy at that time was simple: "Ketchup is not served with french fries." But as they opened more locations in the United States, the demand for ketchup with fries was not going away.

Don and Enid Dunkleman (ironic last name, don'cha think?), who had been McDonald's franchisees from Southern California since 1963, came up with a solution. They created "The Dunk Cup." It was similar to what a small portion of ice cream might be served in today. The Dunk Cups, which had lids, were filled with ketchup in the morning and then refrigerated.

It's kind of hard to believe that at first, they were sold to customers for three or five cents each. Not long after their debut, they became complimentary. The ketchup packets we know today were introduced in 1968 for takeout orders, but Dunk Cups could still be found for many years after that whenever you dined in at a McDonald's.

Chapter 5

BURGER KING

INSTA BURGER KING

In 1953, Keith G. Cramer and his father-in-law, Matthew L. Burns, founded Insta Burger King in Jacksonville, Florida. Keith wasn't new to the food industry; he had some previous restaurant experience. He had once owned Keith's Drive-In Restaurant in Daytona Beach.

One year earlier, Burns had met up with Cramer in California to check out the operation run by the McDonald brothers. While there, they met George Read, the creator of the Insta Broiler and Milkshakes machines.

They decided to enter into a licensing agreement with him in which they would open a McDonald's-type restaurant using his machines to make their burgers and milkshakes. This agreement also allowed them to license the use of the two machines in the State of Florida. Cramer and Burns agreed to give Read a franchise fee along with his profit on the sale of the two machines, plus a share of the two percent royalty fee paid by each prospective franchisee.

The Insta Broiler could not only cook the burger vertically in twelve baskets, each holding up to ten burgers—it would toast the buns at the same time. The buns were placed under the basket that held the burgers, which meant that the drippings would "season" the buns. Read's machine then dropped the cooked patties into "hamburger sauce" made of ketchup, mustard, relish and a special seasoning created by Burns, Cramer, and Read. The sauce was kept warm in a saucepan atop an electric hot plate by the broiler.

Meanwhile, the Insta Milkshake machine flash-froze liquid dairy product to turn into milkshakes. The shakes were so thick that the restaurant had to give everyone a wooden spoon to eat them.

The Insta Broiler did have some problems. The main one was the execution of cooking the burger and the toasted bun. Sometimes the entire restaurant operation came to a halt until the machine could be repaired.

DAVID EDGERTON GETS INVOLVED

A former Howard Johnson's restaurant manager in Miami, Florida, was in Jacksonville looking into a Dairy Queen franchise. David Edgerton was looking for approval from the DQ regional manager to sell burgers on his menu.

While the first "Insta Burger" restaurant (as it was going to be called) was under construction, Burns and Cramer met with Edgerton on a few occasions. Edgerton suggested that they should name it Insta Burger King. He also drew a picture of a king sitting on a hamburger, clutching a milkshake with his arms. Burns and Cramer ended up using both the king design and the new name, which they registered as a trademark and a service mark. The first Insta Burger King building had a twelve-foot pylon facing the front of the building where the king sat on a burger holding his shake.

David Edgerton did not ask for anything in exchange for his ideas. He did, however, end up buying the franchise rights for Dade County, Florida (which included Miami), where Royal Castle had been operating a hamburger empire unopposed since 1938.

He was able to convince the property owner to build out the restaurant, then lease it to him. On March 1, 1954, Edgerton's Insta Burger King opened in Miami. The construction of the building, including a freshly paved parking lot, cost thirteen thousand dollars.

Insta Burger King sold eighteen-cent hamburgers, eighteen-cent milkshakes, ten-cent french fries, and ten-cent soft drinks...and it was averaging less than one hundred dollars a day in sales. It was known as a "self-service drive-in" where you could order from the counter, then take the food to go or eat it in your car. The Miami location featured a first of its kind open-air patio area on the side of the building where you could sit to enjoy your meal.

DAVID MEETS JAMES

During the initial build-out, Edgerton met with James McLamore at the insistence of Miami restaurateur Harvey Fuller. Fuller liked the idea of Insta Burger King but wasn't interested in getting involved with a new concept. James McLamore had sold one of his restaurants, the Colonial Inn, just a few months earlier, so he did have some money stashed away. To be able to join Edgerton on his Insta Burger King crusade, McLamore knew he would also need to sell his Brickell Bridge Restaurant.

Edgerton had invested twenty thousand dollars into the Miami location. Three months later, on June 1, 1954, McLamore joined him and matched the amount. The new corporation, Burger King of Miami, Inc., now had some cash that could be used for expansion.

By the end of 1955, there were four total locations in Miami, all losing money. When 1956 rolled around, not only was McLamore's initial investment gone, but they had assumed new debt. The only way out of this predicament was to find additional investment funds.

McLamore's father-in-law, Dr. Nichol, invested $3,750 for some stock options within the company and loaned them $10,000 at 6 percent. Unfortunately, this alone would not fix the problem. Edgerton and McLamore worked on figuring out the apathetic response that customers had to this new system.

They believed there were multiple causes for the weak sales. First, McLamore and Edgerton could not count on the Insta Machines. They were always breaking down, making it difficult to serve a consistent product. Second, the price for their burgers was eighteen cents, when McDonald's and Royal Castle were at the fifteen-cent price point. As McLamore noted in his autobiography, Insta Burger King was just ordinary and didn't offer anything exceptional.

Dr. Nichol introduced McLamore to Harvey C. Fruehauf, who had recently retired to Miami Beach from Detroit, Michigan. After a lengthy conversation about business, he was offered a 50 percent stake in their corporation in exchange for a $65,000 investment. On April 30, 1956, they closed the deal.

The money was used to build three more restaurant locations. Store number five was selling more than any of the first four spots, but the two newest locations were just as weak on the sales front as the originals. Using the Fruehauf investment to open new stores landed them in an even worse predicament. They were out of money and starting to incur new debt once again.

A WHOPPER OF AN IDEA

On Edgerton and McLamore's trip back from visiting Burns and Cramer in Jacksonville, they stopped into a new Insta Burger King in Gainesville.

The building was a prefab, which meant it could be moved if it didn't do well in its current spot.

After a few hours there, not one customer had walked in. Just down the block, however, customers were lined up at the Whataburger restaurant. The sign outside announced a big hamburger, so McLamore got in line and ordered two burgers. The unwrapped sandwich featured a quarter-pound hamburger patty on a five-inch wide bun topped with lettuce, tomatoes, mayonnaise, pickles, onions, and ketchup. He took one bite and understood the hype. On his walk back to the Insta Burger King, he finished his burger and gave Edgerton the second one. Edgerton liked it too.

On the drive back to Miami, their conversation was all about adding a more massive burger to their menu and then marketing it. They chose the name "Whopper." They decided to add a "Home of the Whopper" sign under the Burger King at all of their locations.

The Whopper—a quarter-pound beef patty topped with mayo, lettuce, tomatoes, pickles, ketchup, and sliced onion on a sesame-seed bun—made its debut at thirty-seven cents. A few weeks later, the price was raised to thirty-nine cents. It was a success from the minute it was added to the menu, and it couldn't have come at a more critical time.

Along with the introduction of the Whopper came the switch to the more reliable Sani-Serve Milkshake machine and a new, improved Insta Broiler machine. Mechanic Karl Sundman had rebuilt the original Insta Broiler machine using an idea from Edgerton. The continuous chain broiler worked much better and became the basis for all future Burger King burger equipment.

McLamore and Edgerton hired Frank Thomas Jr. and Don Thomas of the General Equipment Corporation (GEC) to manufacture the newly dubbed Flame Broiler for all of their current and future locations. GEC liked the machinery so much that they ended up opening a chain of restaurants called Burger Chef.

McLamore and Edgerton let Burns and Cramer know that they had not only replaced the Insta Machines, but that they would be designing their own buildings as well as creating their own operating manuals. The Manual of Operating Data by David Edgerton became the guide to their restaurants. All of the Florida franchises were now looking to them for leadership, too.

WHEN PROBLEMS ARISE, START FRANCHISING

A new obstacle arose: the State of Florida. They had been using a formula given to them by the Sales Tax Department. Three years later, they claimed that their formula was faulty and that the company now owed $8,304. The State of Florida accepted 168 postdated checks to settle the issue. For the next twenty-four months, seven checks would be deposited each month.

Around this time, local businessman Charles Krebs asked if location number five was for sale. Desperate for cash, they could not turn down the twenty thousand dollar offer Krebs made. He agreed to pay a royalty of 2.9 percent a month, and 2 percent of sales would go toward advertising. It was a turning point for the company. They decided to focus their efforts on franchising. Four of their restaurant locations were franchised off, and the money was used to build more franchisable eateries.

Cramer and Burns' franchisees in Broward and Palm Beach were looking to sell. McLamore and Edgerton stepped in to help sell the locations and ended up with a new territorial license that included Broward, Palm Beach, and Monroe counties and a few on the West Coast. They now had exclusive rights to create restaurants in all of South Florida.

Burns and Cramer came to an agreement where Ben Stein, a well-respected businessman in Jacksonville, would come on board as a 50 percent partner and would also lend them money to expand. They tried to emulate the McLamore and Edgerton duo by expanding and adding new stores. But they didn't have the infrastructure for it, and the stores performed poorly. Since they were unable to make payments to Stein on their loan, Stein was forced to take the company from them. He had no experience in this industry and encountered many difficulties when it came to franchising. Stein pushed for McLamore and Edgerton to take over all franchising for the company, something they were seriously considering.

In 1959 Miami's airport was starting to grow, and expanded jet service made the offer more attractive to Edgerton and McLamore. It was more important to them to continue to build profitable South Florida Burger King locations.

CUT OUT THE INSTA AND TAKE CONTROL

By 1961, Ben Stein was at his wit's end with the Burger King franchising situation. He did not have the capacity to execute it properly. He flew to Miami to meet with McLamore to get them to develop the brand nationally.

"Ben, turn over all your rights, title, and interest in the use of the names Burger King, Whopper, and Home of the Whopper, together with your total interest in the trademarks and service marks. With that in hand,

Dave and I will commit to make our best effort to develop Burger King restaurants all over the country and worldwide." recalled James McLamore in his autobiography. "I won't guarantee you a specific performance of any kind because I don't know how successful we will be, but with regard to the royalties, I'll send you 15 percent of anything we collect every month. I can't afford to do any more of [than] that."

Stein agreed. Now that McLamore and Edgerton were in full control, they shortened the name of the restaurants to Burger King.

McLamore and Edgerton decided on a territory-based franchising system as the best way to grow the company quickly. The franchisees were given an exclusive area in which to open a certain number of restaurants. Wilmington, Delaware, was home to the first out of state Burger King store. By 1963, the newly created Whopper College taught and trained franchisees in Edgerton and McLamore's methods.

The jump in the number of store locations made it evident to the duo that they were going to have to take matters into their own hands and manufacture everything that the stores needed. The new manufacturing company was called Davmor Industries, an acronym using Edgerton's first name and James' last name. They began to make hamburger broilers based on Edgerton's 1955 design.

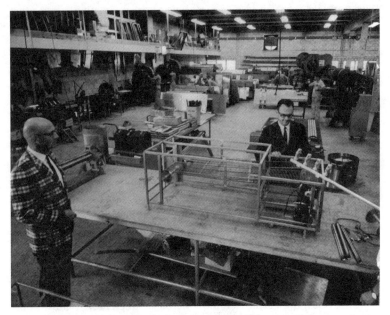

James McLamore looks on as David Edgerton tinkers
with one of their charbroilers.

PILLSBURY BUYS BURGER KING

At this point, many restaurant chains were going public on the stock exchange. Burger King was interested in following suit, but a meeting with the same company that facilitated Howard Johnson's public offering did not turn out as expected. Then their fortunes changed.

On March 26, 1966, the Pillsbury Company contacted them about the possibility of a merger. By August, they had reached an agreement. But two things needed to be taken care of first: the acquisition of the trademarks and the end of the royalty-sharing agreement with Stein.

Pillsbury agreed to pay $2,550,000 to Ben Stein in 1967 to purchase the Burger King trademarks and national franchising rights, along with another $50,000 to cover his lawyer's fees. Pillsbury issued 400,000 shares of common stock and a convertible note worth about $5 million to cover the asking price of $20 million for the 274-unit Burger King company. On January 19, 1967, Burger King and Pillsbury announced the merger, and five months later, the actual merger took place. James McLamore became not only the director of the Burger King company, but also a member of the Pillsbury management team.

And the Whopper was now a whopping forty-five cents.

Initially, Pillsbury allowed Burger King to operate as a separate entity. Over time, Pillsbury made numerous attempts to restructure the company, including cutting back on restaurant expansion. This allowed McDonald's, the leader in the industry, to dominate with a greater number of locations, leaving Burger King a very distant second.

OPERATION PHOENIX

McLamore's reign as director lasted through 1972, when Arthur Rosewall took over. In 1977, due to his declining health, he was replaced by Don Smith, the third highest ranking executive at the McDonald's Corporation.

Smith initiated a plan called "Operation Phoenix" that called for a restructuring of business disciplines, including an update to franchise agreements, standardized restaurant designs, and a menu with a more extensive selection. The newly revamped menu would include chicken and fish sandwiches as well as breakfast.

The Burger King Kingdom was then created to compete with the McDonald's McDonaldland juggernaut, which had kids hooked. The Kingdom featured the Magical Burger King, the Duke of Doubt, Sir Shake-A-Lot, the Burger Thing, and the Wizard of Fries. By 1989, most of the characters were phased out, except for the Burger King, who would return as "The King" in a series of slightly creepy and entertaining commercials in 2003.

After Smith ended territorial franchises in 1979, the proportion of company owned restaurants rose from 8 percent to 42 percent. Company sales also rose by 15 percent in 1980. Shortly after that, Smith was snapped up by PepsiCo. The good news was short-lived, as sales began to decline after his departure.

FIRST SHOTS FIRED

Pillsbury's executive vice president of restaurant operations, Norman E. Brinker, was given the unenviable task of trying to turn around Burger King's fortunes. His main initiative was a series of commercials where Burger King attacked competitors, kicking off the famous Burger Wars of the 1980s.

But Brinker was not able to turn the company around, and in 1989, Grand Metropolitan purchased Pillsbury. By 2002, the company became independent again after a group of investment firms led by TPG bought them out. Within four years, they took the company public.

There was a period where the changes brought on by the new company had sales on the upswing. But by 2010, things were beginning to look grim. Then 3G Capital of Brazil stepped in and purchased Burger King for $3.26 billion. The Burger King stock listed on the New York Stock Exchange was removed immediately.

3G merged Burger King with Tim Hortons in August 2014. The newly formed company, now known as Restaurant Brands International, added Popeyes Louisiana Kitchen to the portfolio in March, 2017. Burger King now boasts almost 17,000 locations with over 1.2 billion dollars in sales.

BURGER KING'S QUIRKY TRADEMARK ISSUES

Burger King Drive Inn of Alberta, Canada

Burger King Drive Inn was a mini-chain of restaurants founded in 1956 in Alberta, Canada. They also featured Kentucky Fried Chicken until about 1979, when their licensing agreement expired. The restaurants were sold in 1990, but founders William R. Jarvis and James Duncan Rae kept the "Burger King" trademark. The "Burger King" name was sold to the Burger King company by Jarvis and Rae in 1985 for one million dollars. The company wasted no time in announcing that there would soon be Burger King restaurants in Alberta.

Burger King of Mattoon, Illinois

When Edgerton and McLamore's Burger King decided to open their first location in the state of Illinois in 1961, little did they know the can of worms that they were opening. Since 1952, Gene and Betty Hoots had owned Frigid Queen. In 1954, they expanded their menu to include hamburgers and fries, among other foods. The name of the restaurant was changed to Burger King in 1957, and in 1959, the name was registered as a state trademark in Illinois.

By 1967, the number of corporate Burger King locations was hovering around fifty, and the couple decided to take a stand. They brought a lawsuit against Burger King of Florida in 1968, believing that their state trademark gave them the exclusive rights to the name of Burger King in the state of Illinois.

BK of Florida argued that their federal trademark superseded the couple's state trademark. The court decision gave the Hoots exclusive rights to an area within a twenty-mile radius from the location of their restaurant, and Burger King of Florida the rights everywhere else.

Gene and Betty Hoots are now retired. The Burger King of Mattoon was sold to Cory Sanders. Thirty years later, the closest corporate Burger King location is in Tuscola, Illinois, twenty-five miles away.

Hungry Jack's of Australia

There is only one country in the world where Burger King does not operate under their name, and that is Australia. In 1971, when Burger King was establishing itself down under, they learned that their name had already been trademarked. They gave their Australian franchisee Jack Cowin a list of possible new names from Burger King and Pillsbury's already registered trademarks. He chose the name used by Pillsbury's US pancake mix, Hungry Jack. The only change he made was to add an apostrophe-s.

Whopper Burger in San Antonio, Texas

In 1955 Frank Bates founded Whopper Burger in San Antonio, Texas. He was the owner of the rights to the name "Whopper," which effectively kept Burger King from using the name there. Burger King did open a store in the area for a brief time and renamed their signature sandwich as the Deluxe. The store did not survive.

Fast forward to 1983, when Bates passed away and his wife sold the restaurant chain to a couple of Burger King franchisees a year later, who in turn sold it to the Burger King company. All of the Whopper Burger locations were converted to Burger Kings in 1985, and at last, the people of San Antonio could finally enjoy a real deal Whopper.

Chapter

6

WENDY'S

Before we delve into the history of Wendy's, I need to give some you Kentucky Fried Chicken history. Again, I know this is a book about burgers, but it's all going to make sense.

THE COLONEL KNOWS BEST

Phil Clauss was the owner of multiple locations of the Hobby House restaurant. His head cook at the Fort Wayne location was a gentleman by the name of Dave Thomas, who had recently returned to work after a three-year stint in the Army in 1953. Thomas met eighteen-year-old waitress Lorraine Buskirk that same year, and they were wed in 1954.

Dave Thomas was eventually promoted to vice president of not only the Hobby House but of a new barbecue restaurant called the Hobby Ranch House. It was then that Clauss told Thomas about an interesting character named Colonel Harland Sanders whom he had met at a restaurant convention in 1956. The Colonel had a white mustache and goatee, walked with a gold-tipped cane, and drove a white Cadillac.

Sanders pitched his now world-famous secret herbs and spices along with a more efficient way to fry chicken. In the 1950s, there were no KFC stand-alone restaurants; his chicken was just a featured item on other menus. The Colonel would sell you his spice blend and pressure cookers to cook the chicken. He would make a nickel per piece of chicken sold in perpetuity.

Dave Thomas was not sold on the idea until he realized that the method significantly cut the prep time for fried chicken. The public also seemed interested in it. So Clauss agreed to add Kentucky Fried Chicken to his menus at his Fort Wayne location and others throughout the Midwest.

Throughout the next few years, Thomas' relationship with the Colonel grew, and he considered the Colonel a mentor. In 1960, Clauss opened up four Kentucky Fried Chicken franchises in Columbus, Ohio. One year later, sales were horrible. So Clauss offered Thomas the opportunity to turn them around. Thomas was guaranteed a forty percent ownership stake in the company once he paid off the original $250,000 investment. Clauss and Lorraine had faith in him, but the Colonel, not so much.

"Listen to the Colonel, boy," the Colonel told Thomas, according to his autobiography. "As your friend, get out now—while you can. Things are just too far gone here."

In 1962, when Thomas arrived in Columbus to turn the stores around, things were even worse than he thought. None of the locations had any credit, he discovered, and even his friend Colonel Sanders required cash on delivery for any purchases.

Thomas spruced up all four spots with a brand-new coat of paint and created the wobbling or rotating (depending on how you look at it) red and white bucket sign featuring Colonel Sanders' face on it. He shrank the menu and focused on fried chicken. There was no money for advertising, so he exchanged chicken for airtime on local TV and radio stations. Thomas also convinced his chicken supplier to pay for a newspaper ad.

All his ideas and hard work paid off. In 1968, the four locations were sold. He pocketed $1.5 million for his forty percent, which would amount to just under eleven million dollars today. At the age of thirty-five, Dave Thomas was now a millionaire.

MILLIONAIRES DON'T SIT AROUND

Dave Thomas didn't sit around and enjoy his success. He was cooking up an idea around his love of hamburgers. He mentioned what was rolling around in his head to his friend Len Immke. Immke told him it was hard to get a good lunch in downtown Columbus. Immke suggested that Thomas should consider opening his new restaurant in one of the buildings that he owned on Broad Street.

The fast food scene was moving away from quality and toward a 'profits first' mentality. Thomas was interested in turning things around by focusing on quality and an old-school restaurant atmosphere. There were Tiffany-style lamps and bentwood chairs, and there was turn of the century advertising on the tops of all the tables.

Part of what inspired Dave Thomas was Kewpee Hamburgers and their square burgers and thick malt shakes. He liked how the corners stuck out of the buns—customers could see the quality of the meat.

The menu was simple, one of the takeaways from his time spent revamping Clauss' restaurants. It featured made-to-order single, double, and triple hamburgers, along with their "Secret Recipe" chili, french fries, soft drinks, and their dairy dessert, the Frosty.

Dave Thomas was adamant about the consistency of the Frosty. Thicker than a milkshake and not as firm as soft-serve ice cream, it had to be eaten with a spoon. The original Frosty was a mixture of chocolate and vanilla. Thomas thought chocolate was too strong and would overwhelm the burgers.

WENDA'S

Dave Thomas wanted to convey a wholesome image for his restaurant, so he named it after his redheaded, freckle-faced eight-year-old daughter Melinda Lou Thomas. As a toddler, she had struggled to pronounce Melinda, so her family called her "Wenda." The restaurant would be called Wendy's, since Wenda's didn't quite have the right ring to it.

Thomas was heavily criticized by the media for moving into the overcrowded fast food space. At the very least, he hoped to provide a summer job for his kids.

On November 15, 1969, Wendy's held its grand opening in downtown Columbus. Wenda—well, let's just call her Wendy from now on—was walking around charming everyone in the signature blue and white striped dress that has now been made world famous by the image of Wendy in the logo.

One year later, the second Wendy's opened in Columbus; it featured an industry innovation. While drive-thrus were beginning to become popular, Wendy's pick-up window featured an entirely separate grill just for those orders, which sped up wait times.

A SERIES OF FIRSTS

In 1972, they hit the Ohio TV airwaves with a series of commercials featuring their "Quality Is Our Recipe" slogan and an animated Wendy dancing with hamburgers.

And in August 1972, the first Wendy's franchise opened, owned by L.S. Hartzog. He went on to open his restaurants in the area of Indianapolis,

Indiana. Soon Wendy's began enlisting new franchise owners at an unprecedented rate for such a new restaurant.

One of those franchise owners was Jim Near, a friend of Dave Thomas' from his Kentucky Fried Chicken days. He was the owner of a rival down the street back then, Burger Boy Food-A-Rama. Near later became vice president of that company and an executive at Borden Inc. when they bought out Burger Boy. In 1974, he became a Wendy's franchise owner and went on to own thirty-eight more locations in West Virginia and Florida.

After he sold his locations back to the Wendy's corporation in 1978, Jim Near established the Sisters Chicken & Biscuits chain. Sisters became a division of Wendy's in 1981 and then was sold off in 1987 to their largest franchise owner.

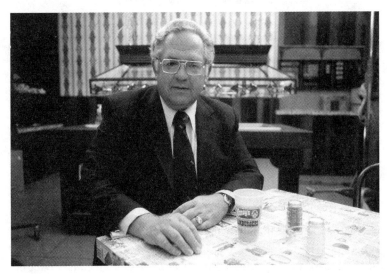

Late 1970s: Dave Thomas sitting at a newspaper print table inside of a Wendy's restaurant.

Wendy's initial public stock offering in September 1976 on the NASDAQ exchange was for one million common shares of stock at twenty-eight dollars per share.

In March 1978, Wendy's opened its thousandth restaurant in Springfield, Tennessee, setting an industry record. By November 1980, they were at two thousand locations.

Wendy's seemed to be on a roll. Then, in 1982, Dave Thomas retired. Store sales then flattened out, and the company was struggling in the dog-eat-dog fast-food market.

HELLO, CLARA

Everything changed on January 10, 1984, when elderly actress and former manicurist Clara Peller, along with Elizabeth Shaw and Mildred Lane, were featured in the uber-successful "Where's the Beef?" commercial. Peller went on to star in ten commercials for Wendy's. The "Where's the Beef?" campaign was such a juggernaut that it spawned an entire line of merchandise, from puffy stickers and puzzles to trash cans.

The original commercial registered the highest consumer awareness level in the advertising industry's history. The original "Where's the Beef?" ad was voted the most popular commercial in the United States in 1984.

In 1985, Clara Peller appeared in a thirty-second TV commercial for Prego spaghetti sauce where, alluding to her now famous catchphrase, she said, "I found it!" "I really found it!" "I finally found it!" and "Boy, did I find it!" This did not sit well with the folks at Wendy's. Peller was fired, and a Wendy's spokesperson issued this statement:

"The commercial infers that Clara found the beef at somewhere other than Wendy's restaurants. Unfortunately, Clara's appearance in the ads makes it extremely difficult for her to serve as a credible spokesperson for our products."

BRING IN JIM NEAR AND HIS RIGHT-HAND MAN

The sales for 1985 were incredible. But the company got complacent and made some mistakes, including an ill-fated attempt to penetrate the breakfast market. By the end of the year, 20 percent of the company's stores were on the verge of bankruptcy.

Dave Thomas suggested that his old buddy Jim Near take on the job of president and chief operating officer. Near agreed to the position on one condition: Thomas had to return to active duty as the face for Wendy's new advertising campaign.

Near also wanted Dave Thomas to become a traveling mentor for the company. Thomas taught Wendy's franchises that everyone needed to have an MBA, "Mop Bucket Attitude." When he wasn't visiting stores, he was filming commercials. Thomas appeared in more than eight hundred of them and in turn became a household name.

Near refined and standardized Wendy's operating model. Six years after his changes, the employee turnover rate had dropped to 20 percent from 55 percent. Wendy's then saw sixteen years of same-store sales increases. The creation of the 99 cent menu in 1988 and the Wendy's Super Value Menu in 1989 with nine items at 99 cents turned the fast-food market on its ear.

If there was any doubt that the company had turned the corner, the earnings for 1995 were above Wendy's previous earnings peak in 1985. Unfortunately, the following year, Near died of a heart attack while at the Olympic Games in Atlanta.

Dave Thomas passed away from cancer on January 8, 2002, at his home in Fort Lauderdale, Florida, at sixty-nine and was buried in his hometown of Columbus. In 2006, Wendy's moved their headquarters to Dublin, Ohio.

CHANGES ABOUND

Wendy Thomas followed in her father's footsteps, making her Wendy's advertisement debut in a series of commercials that began to air on TV in November 2010. Two years later, Morgan Smith Goodwin took over as a Wendy-like character in a series of commercials with the slogan, "Now that's better."

In late 2011, the recipe for Wendy's burger patty used in the single, double, and triple hamburgers was altered. The new Dave's Hot 'N Juicy hamburger patty was thicker. The iconic square shape was slightly rounded off on the corners. Red onions replaced white, and the condiments ketchup and mayonnaise made the cut while mustard got the heave-ho.

Now at well over 6,500 locations, Wendy's continues the philosophy set forth by Dave Thomas, "Quality is our recipe."

WENDY'S QUIRKY FACTS

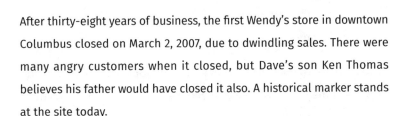

After thirty-eight years of business, the first Wendy's store in downtown Columbus closed on March 2, 2007, due to dwindling sales. There were many angry customers when it closed, but Dave's son Ken Thomas believes his father would have closed it also. A historical marker stands at the site today.

There was only one Frosty machine at the first Wendy's location. Dave Thomas would mix the chocolate and vanilla ice cream himself.

When Thomas' mentor "Colonel" Harland Sanders passed away on December 16, 1980, he ordered flags at all of the Wendy's locations to fly at half-staff.

The "sisters" in the Wendy's-founded Sisters Chicken and Biscuits restaurant chain refers to Dave Thomas' other three daughters.

After Thomas returned to the company in the late 1980s, his new business card read, "Founder and Jim's Right-Hand Man," in reference to his good friend Jim Near.

When he was just fifteen years old, Dave Thomas dropped out of high school. It was a decision that haunted him until he decided to finish his high school education in 1993. Thomas was sixty-one years old. He had always felt that education was an essential part of the formative years and did not want to send the wrong message to everyone, especially children. Thomas received his GED from Coconut Creek High School near Fort Lauderdale, Florida. He was voted "Most Likely to Succeed" by the senior class, and he and his wife Lorraine were named the school's prom king and queen for that year.

In 1994, the city of Philadelphia wanted to fine Wendy's $98,400, claiming the restaurant was shorting their quarter-pound burgers by up to a quarter of an ounce. Philly later announced that they had made a mistake and withdrew the fine.

In 2000, Dave Thomas was recognized in the *Guinness Book of World Records* as the founder who has made the most television commercial appearances as a spokesperson for his company.

Close to three hundred million Frostys are served annually at Wendy's. The Frosty must be served at a temperature of between nineteen and twenty-one degrees to keep the right amount of thickness and texture.

Chapter

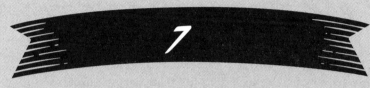

7

BURGER WARS

The Burger Wars between Burger King, McDonald's, and Wendy's from 1982 to 1985 were never really about who had the best food. They were more about one-upping and outsmarting the competition on the advertising front. It was also the battle for the number two burger spot in the United States, as McDonald's had a commanding lead and firm grip on the number one spot.

WHO THREW THAT FIRST STONE?

We can track the beginnings of the Burger Wars to when Burger King lured away Don Smith, McDonald's third highest ranking exec, in 1977. His "Operation Phoenix" began the head-to-head competition between BK and McDonald's. After his departure in 1980, Burger King sales were suffering, and Norman E. Brinker from BK's parent company started a series of commercials that went after their competitors.

In September, 1982, Burger King cast the first stone with a twenty-million-dollar series of national TV commercials that featured five-year-old Sarah Michelle Gellar, who would later become famous for playing the lead in *Buffy the Vampire Slayer*.

A VERY BIG MESSAGE COMMERCIAL:

"When I order a regular burger at McDonald's, they make it with 20 percent less meat than Burger King. Unbelievable! Luckily, I know the perfect way to show McDonald's how I feel. I go to Burger King."

BROILING VERSUS FRYING COMMERCIAL:

"I can't figure McDonald's out. Everybody knows flame
broiling beats frying three to one. It was on TV. But
McDonald's is frying their hamburgers, unbelievable!
Well, I like them flame broiled, so what are you gonna
do? I know, go to Burger King!"

Other commercials featured Elisabeth Shue of *Back to the Future*,
Adventures in Babysitting, and *Leaving Las Vegas* fame.

A FRIENDLY WAGER COMMERCIAL:

"Stop what you're doing and go to your phone. I
wanna make a bet with you. See, in a coast-to-coast
survey, three out of four people said they liked their
burgers fixed their way. That's how we do it at Burger
King. Now here's the bet, pick up your phone and call
any four people. I'll bet at least three will choose to
have it your way like at Burger King. Any takers?"

A VERY IMPORTANT MESSAGE COMMERCIAL:

"At this time, we'd like to offer our sympathy to
McDonald's and Wendy's. You see, the Whopper beat
the Big Mac for best taste overall among consumers
of both burgers. In a similar test, we beat Wendy's
Single. Now, that may have surprised McDonald's
and Wendy's, so we just wanted to say, it's OK, guys,
winning isn't everything, but it sure is fun!"

LAWSUITS, HERE WE COME

McDonald's tried to prevent the commercials from airing by having their lawyers file an injunction. McDonald's then made sure to sneak in a jab at Burger King at the hearing: "The representation[s] that Burger King's hamburger sandwiches are broiled while McDonald's are fried...are false and misleading because Burger King burgers are often steamed and then reheated or warmed in microwave ovens before sales to consumers." Ouch.

The lawsuit didn't deter Burger King from continuing with their series of ads. Another commercial preached that if you came to BK and said, "The Whopper beats the Big Mac," you'd get a free hamburger with every one ordered.

While McDonald's was in legal mode, Wendy's publicly asked Burger King and McDonald's to participate in a nationwide taste test conducted by an independent party. They both ignored the request.

Wendy's joined the wars on September 30, 1982, by filing their own injunction to stop the ads, asking for twenty-five million dollars in damages. Both McDonald's and Wendy's believed that the ads were misleading and wanted Burger King to reveal precisely how their taste tests were done and to issue corrective ads. Wendy's chairman Robert L. Barney called Burger King's claims an insult to Wendy's customers.

On October 29, 1982, the big three reached an uneasy truce. McDonald's and Wendy's would not soldier on with their lawsuits as long as Burger King submitted a schedule for the removal of the ads. It appeared that Burger King had agreed with its initial public statement: "The comparative commercials were to be of short duration. The purpose has been served, and they are being phased out."

Then, later that same day, Burger King released a new statement: "The campaign of comparative commercials has served its purpose. The commercials will be gradually replaced over the next several weeks, and the campaign was planned to be of short duration anyway."

A few days later, they were back at it again over Burger King's public statements. Burger King's newest statement clarified that only one of the controversial commercials would continue to run through the end of the year.

It didn't stop Burger King from running full page newspaper ads on November 17 that proclaimed in giant lettering: "GUESS WHO WON..." and said, "The Whopper beat the Big Mac and Wendy's Single" and "Broiling beat frying."

The next bit of the burger war falls into the *What were they thinking?* category. On November 20, 1982, a rogue Burger King restaurant owner in Tampa Bay took the Burger Wars into his own hands. "Burger King Wins the Battle of the Burgers" was written in red on one of the glass doors at the establishment, but it didn't end there. They took a life-size Ronald McDonald doll and placed him in a coffin, then put a wooden stake through his stomach. A note on the coffin said, "They got me in the McRibs." Right next to Ronald was a Magical Burger King proclaiming, "The Whopper Whips Wendy's Singles" and "Winners Served Here." Neither McDonald's nor Burger King corporate were happy about the stunt.

Burger King finished up the year with "Have yourself a merry little Christmas" commercial, featuring a very young Sarah Michelle Gellar, Lea Thompson (Marty's mom in *Back to the Future*), and Elisabeth Shue. Near the end of the commercial, Gellar zings 'em with a "Merry Christmas, McDonald's" comment. It should be of no surprise that Burger King sales were up 13 percent by the end of 1982.

YEAR TWO STARTS SLOW

The year 1983 started quietly until Burger King released five commercials, all revolving around broiling versus frying.

Elisabeth Shue opens up with "Burger King would like to suggest that everyone from McDonald's please leave the room..." she says. The commercial went on to point out that in a coast-to-coast opinion poll, broiling beat frying nearly three to one.

By September, Wendy's unleashed commercials with the same satirical tone that they would perfect in 1984. In obvious digs at McDonald's and Burger King, two memorable spots started with: "Two famous hamburger places use frozen hamburgers," and "At some hamburger places, when you order special toppings, they say you'll have to wait."

Meanwhile, Burger King's newest ads, also in September, featured the "MacDonalds" family, which, of course, were in no way related to their rival McDonald's. In one ad, the five family members, wearing cheesy fake glasses with attached oversized noses and mustaches, explain what made them switch to Burger King. The narrator of the ad says, "OK, America, now when you switch to Burger King, you can tell 'em..." and here's the clincher, the family removes their disguises and say in chorus, "The MacDonalds sent you!"

Before we move on into the 1984 portion of the Burger Wars, let's consider how many locations each of the big three had at the time. McDonald's had approximately 6,100 stores. Burger King was in second place with 3,320, and Wendy's had 2,650 restaurants. In 1983, the big three spent more than $318 million on television commercials, which, believe it or not, only accounted for 3 percent of their total annual sales.

Burger King started strong in January of 1984 by cutting the price of its hamburger by about 35 percent to thirty-nine cents for a limited time. McDonald's matched it for a short time in a few select New York cities. Wendy's smallest burger was a quarter-pound, so they didn't get involved with the temporary price drops.

An event unrelated to the Burger Wars, but a vital burger history note nonetheless, was the death of Ray Kroc, founder of the McDonald's Corporation, on January 14, 1984, at the age of eighty-one. The day after his passing, all flags at McDonald's were flown at half-staff. Burger King cofounder James McLamore had "great respect and admiration" for Ray Kroc, and Wendy's founder Dave Thomas hailed Kroc as a "trailblazer and an outstanding American."

WHERE'S THE BEEF?

The most iconic commercials to come out of the Burger Wars were the ads of the "Where's the Beef?" ad campaign, an eight-million-dollar series of ads created by Dancer Fitzgerald Sample. Along with the TV spots, Wendy's also distributed two million "competitive meat detectors," which were small magnifying glasses with a printed advisory to use at restaurants other than Wendy's to locate the meat.

"Fluffy Bun" was directed by Joe Sedelmaier and featured senior citizen Clara Peller saying the now-legendary phrase, "Where's the Beef?" The original ad showed a young couple ordering a burger and mentioning the giant fluffy bun. After lifting the top bun, it would reveal the small beef patty. It just didn't work.

The revamped idea had three little old ladies replacing the young couple at the "Home of the Big Bun" with Clara Peller delivering the memorable catchphrase: "Where's the Beef?" Clara was supposed to say, "Where is all the beef?" but her emphysema prevented her from uttering the entire phrase.

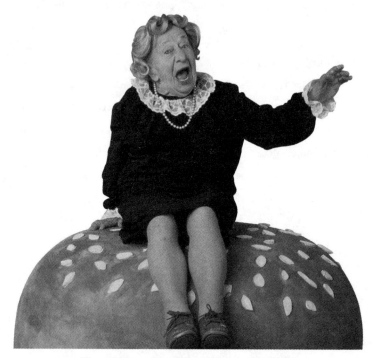

Clara Peller, star of the Where's the Beef?
Commercials.

The fluffy bun was followed by a similar ad that ends with Clara at a Big Bun talking on the phone, and another where she's driving erratically with two other ladies sitting in the back seat. She ends up driving under a golden arch on her way to multiple drive-thru windows, each of which slams shut before she can place her order.

The one-two punch of the ridiculous looking tiny patty sitting inside of a massive burger bun, with Peller just short of yelling the beef line, was perfect. I distinctly remember the popularity of these ads but didn't realize they only ran for a few months.

"Where's the Beef?" crossed over into the pop culture lexicon, and so did Peller's likeness. You could find merchandise like puffy stickers, posters, mugs, T-shirts, and garbage cans for sale everywhere.

Clara Peller made it to the cover of the May-June 1984 issue of *Consumer's Digest*. Over the next few years, she made appearances at Wrestlemania II, in the film *Moving Violations*, and in the aforementioned Prego Plus spaghetti sauce commercial.

The strangest use of the phrase came during the 1984 presidential primary debate when Democratic candidate Walter Mondale used "Where's the Beef?" about rival candidate Gary Hart's previous comments.

A little-known fact about this series of commercials is that there was an earlier and much less memorable version featuring an older gentleman saying, "Where's the beef?" while waiting in line at "Whopping Big Burger."

By November, 1984, Burger King was cooking up a series of new ads aimed at McDonald's that ended with the phrase, "You'll never have to eat a fried quarter pounder again." Wendy's also went after McDonald's, but this time they targeted their Chicken McNuggets.

The "Where's the Beef?" phenomenon caused a downturn in Whopper sales. Burger King responded in May 1985 by increasing the size of their Whopper from 3.6 ounces to 4.2 ounces. The Whopper was changed to a Kaiser-like roll, reducing the bun to 4½ inches in diameter, down from 5 inches. The TV ads to support the more massive Whopper featured celebrities like Mr. T, Oakland Raiders defensive end Lyle Alzado, and Emmanuel Lewis of "Webster."

MCDLT HISTORY

The most infamous sandwich in the Burger Wars was McDonald's McDLT. It was the creation of a pair of McDonald's franchisees from Cleveland, Ohio, brothers Nick and Gus Karos. The first Lettuce & Tomato Special, or LTS, as it was known initially, came with pickles, onions, ketchup, iceberg lettuce, mayonnaise, tomato, and cheese on a quarter-pound patty, not too different from you might find at any spot that specializes in burgers nowadays.

What made it special was the packaging. It was thought up by Will May, a McDonald's franchisee from Shreveport, Louisiana. The two-section Styrofoam container kept the top bun with all of the toppings cool, while the right side of the container held the bottom bun and burger patty, which were kept hot.

The first LTS was sold on January 2, 1984. In the fall of 1984, McDonald's began testing the LTS in select markets. By February, 1985, they were in forty locations, with plans to expand to four hundred restaurants the following month.

When it finally launched nationwide in early November, 1985, it had already been renamed the McDLT. But it was never able to live up to the hype that McDonald's had given it. The sandwich could have stood on its own merits but was saddled with that bad gimmicky Styrofoam container, which to this day is what most folks remember. Well, that and the Jason Alexander (Seinfeld) musical McDLT commercial, which is hard to erase from your memory.

BURGER KING BACK AT IT

By early January of 1986, Burger King had released a newspaper ad that said:

> *"Lettuce & tomato, what on earth is so new? We've done it for years. And made it special for you. Flame Broiling's the difference. And there's only one place for the Burger King Whopper with that flame broiled taste!"*
>
> *"...AND WE'LL ALSO ACCEPT ALL McDLT COUPONS."*

The worst commercial campaign during the Burger Wars had to be Burger King's series of ads featuring Herb, the last person in the US to have not eaten a burger from Burger King. The ads and TV commercials revolved around trying to convince Herb to come in for a burger. His identity was eventually revealed during the 1986 Super Bowl.

The first person to spot Herb at a BK would receive five thousand dollars, and every person in the restaurant at that time would be entered in a drawing to win one million dollars. Later, you could grab a 99 cent Whopper by going into Burger King and saying, "I'm not Herb." The problem with the promotion was that no one ever really cared about Herb's predicament. It died a quick death.

After skipping out on the meat and potatoes part of the Burger Wars, Hardee's jumped into the battle during September, 1985, just as it was winding down among the big three.

Hardee's ads slowly trickled out over the next year touting their new quarter-pound burgers, burgers that were "thicker and juicier than Burger King, Wendy's, or McDonald's." By March, 1987, Hardee's felt they should be considered one of the big three in the hamburger world. They released two notable commercials, the latter of which was a direct jab at Burger King.

The commercial featured a Burger King-ish magician with a crown making a burger shrink in size. This dig was about Burger King's larger Whopper, which had been was advertised in May, 1985. The Whopper had undergone some changes since then and was no longer 4.2 ounces.

On May 6, 1987, the *Los Angeles Times* ran a story about restaurants looking for a piece of the forty-eight-billion-dollar burger market. The source for the information was *Restaurant Business* magazine, which estimated that McDonald's sales made up 37 percent of the market, while Burger King was at 16 percent and Wendy's at 10 percent, leaving 37 percent for every other restaurant to battle over.

In 1987, McDonald's continued its dominance, while Burger King ended up laying off 15 percent of its workforce. Wendy's also reported its first operating loss since they opened in 1969. It was not a good year for two of the big three, but they would bounce back.

It was silent for quite a bit, and then...

BURGER WARS PART DEUX

On August 26, 2015, Burger King took out full-page ads in the *Chicago Tribune* and *New York Times* directed at McDonald's. In the "open letter," Burger King proposed a collaboration for Peace Day called the "McWhopper." The idea was to combine parts of two of the restaurants' signature burgers. There was also a website with a plan for the product and uniform packaging for the McWhopper.

The McWhopper would be served at a one-time pop-up in Atlanta, Georgia, on September 21, Peace Day. Atlanta was the chosen city, as it was a middle point between McDonald's HQ in Oak Brook, Illinois, and Burger King's in Miami, Florida.

McDonald's turned down the offer. McDonald's CEO Steve Easterbrook said, "We love the intention but think our two brands could do something bigger to make a difference."

On September 1, 2015, Burger King announced that the Peace Day Burger would feature ingredients from Denny's, Giraffas, Krystal, Wayback Burgers, and, of course, Burger King.

The Burger Wars were a golden era for advertising in the hamburger industry along with significant sales increases not likely to be seen again. I want to think there's another big burger war on the horizon, but it's not likely to happen. Luckily, we are left with memorable catchphrases like "Where's the Beef?" and not-so-memorable campaigns like "Herb." But in the end, the consumer won as the big three had to put their best foot forward.

Chapter

8

BURGER RESTAURANTS

Burger restaurants that have shut down live on in the memories of their loyal customers. Here are some restaurants that have left us and some that have stood the test of time.

Arctic Circle

Year Founded: *1950*
City Founded: *Salt Lake City, Utah*
Type: *Regional*
Founder: *Don Carlos Edwards*
Number of Locations at the Chain's Peak: *308*
Locations Still in Operation: *63*
Slogan: *"Take Home A Bagful"*

Don Carlos Edwards was not a newbie to the food scene. In the 1920s, Don had sold food via a trailer at carnivals and fairs. In 1941, he opened up the Don Carlos Bar-Be-Q restaurant. When he went to open a second location nine years later, he opened the first Arctic Circle in Salt Lake City, Utah, instead.

Don created a signature sauce that was initially intended for his burgers. This pink sauce consisted of ketchup, mayonnaise, some garlic, and a few other spices. After inadvertently dipping a fry in the sauce, he realized it was really meant for fried spuds.

Arctic Circle also lays claim to having invented the kid's meal. Back in the 1950s, they would add a toy and special box to any food ordered for a child.

Bell's Burger/Taco Bell

Year Founded: *1950*
City Founded: *San Bernardino, California*
Type: *Worldwide*
Founder: *Glen Bell*
Number of Locations: *currently over 7,000*
Slogan: *"Think outside the bun."*

When you think of Taco Bell, hamburgers are not the first thing that comes to mind. Glen Bell originally opened a hot dog drive-in in 1948. In 1950, he followed it with a burger stand when the McDonald's phenomenon was starting to spread. Everyone else had the same idea, so he switched concepts to tacos. It seems like it worked out for him in the end.

Burger Boy Food-O-Rama/ Borden Burger

Year Founded: *1961*
City Founded: *Columbus, Ohio*
Type: *Regional*
Founders: *Milton O. Lustnauer and Roy Tuggle*
Number of Locations at the Chain's Peak: *48*
Locations Still in Operation: *None*
Slogan: *"Bigger Better Faster"*

Burger Boy Food-A-Rama is remembered fondly for its Whirling Satellite sign, which could be seen from miles away. BBF's vice president, Jim Near, would later play an integral part in preventing Wendy's from going out of business in the 1980s.

In 1969, Burger Boy Food-O-Rama was sold to Borden and changed its name to Borden Burger BBF (Borden Better Foods). By the mid-1970s, most of the locations had closed up shop.

Burger Castle

Year Founded: *1964*
City Founded: *Hialeah, Florida*
Type: *Regional*
Founder: *Charles Edwards Krebs*
Number of Locations at the Chain's Peak: *35*
Locations Still in Operation: *None*
Slogan: *"Home of the Giant"*

Charles Krebs became the first franchisee for the Burger King chain in South Florida in 1957. Because of their tumultuous relationship, Burger King would not allow Mr. Krebs to open a second Burger King. So he did the next best thing. He created his own chain called Burger Castle. The first location would open in Hialeah, Florida, on July 10, 1964.

The layout of the restaurant was exactly like a Burger King of that era. The outside featured a giant twenty-one-foot sign in the shape of a king-type character with a crown on his head holding a shake in one hand and a hamburger in the other.

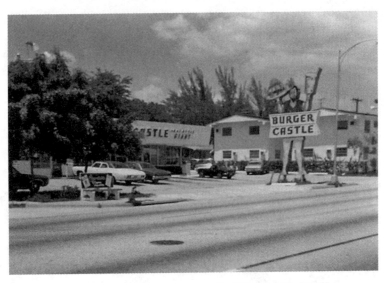

Burger Castle with the twenty-one-foot Giant outside in 1972 in Miami, Florida.

The menu consisted of the "Flavor-Broiled" Giant Burger (similar to Burger King's Whopper, which was topped with tomatoes, lettuce, pickles, ketchup and mayo), a regular burger, fries, shakes, and soft drinks.

On September 18, 1968, Krebs' neighbor and friend W.J. Fowler purchased Burger Castle from him. W.J. Fowler added a commissary for production, and after a lawsuit by Burger King, changed the logo from the king to a knight with a shield. New additions to the menu were fried chicken, a roast beef sandwich, and a filet of fish sandwich.

Burger Castle had locations in Connecticut, Florida, Illinois, Indiana, Louisiana, Maryland, North Carolina, Rhode Island, South Carolina, and Wisconsin. Twenty restaurants were in South Florida, which makes sense since their headquarters were located in Miami, Florida.

In the early 1970s, there was a push to expand into California, but it did not come to pass. By the middle of the 1970s, most of their restaurants were gone. The only remnant left of Burger Castle is the bottom half of the twenty-one-foot sign, still up at their old location in Perrine, Florida.

Burger Chef

Year Founded: *1957*
City Founded: *Indianapolis, Indiana*
Type: *Nationwide*
Founders: *brothers Donald and Frank Thomas*
Number of Locations at the Chain's Peak: *1,200*
Locations Still in Operation: *None*
Signature Burgers: *Big Chef and Super Chef*
Slogan: *"There's more to like at Burger Chef"*

Burger King had hired the General Restaurant Equipment company to build a broiler for them. Inspired by BK, General Restaurant Equipment saw the potential in starting their own burger chain. The first step was to design and create their own broiler to cook burgers. They even went so far as to advertise their first location as "Indianapolis' first Florida-style self-service drive-in!" in the Indianapolis News on March 24, 1957.

In just ten years, Burger Chef became the second largest burger chain, with only about one hundred fewer locations than McDonald's. General Foods Corporation purchased the Burger Chef chain in 1968, which helped to fund its rapid expansion. Under General Foods, they reached their peak of 1,200 locations in 1972.

Burger Chef's mascots were Burger Chef and his younger sidekick Jeff. Burger Chef's Funmeal, which debuted in 1973, featured Burger Chef and Jeff as well as Burgerini, Count Fangburger, Burgerilla, and Cackleburger.

Each Funmeal cardboard box included riddles and puzzles galore and a small toy. McDonald's later introduced their Happy Meal, a similar concept. Burger Chef sued them in 1979 but ultimately lost the $5.5 million lawsuit.

The late 1970s and early 1980s were not kind to Burger Chef as they struggled financially. In 1982, the 679 locations of Burger Chef (420 of which were franchised) were purchased by Hardee's for forty-four million dollars. Many Burger Chef locations were converted to Hardee's, while franchises or restaurants near pre-existing Hardee's were allowed to switch to a different brand altogether.

Some independent Burger Chefs continued to operate for years after the Hardee's purchase. The last Burger Chef restaurant, which was in Cookeville, Tennessee, closed when its franchise agreement expired in 1996. For those of you still longing for a Burger Chef fix, Hardee's has been known to bring back the Big Chef from time to time at some of their Midwestern locations.

You can see a Burger Chef restaurant in action on season seven of the TV show *Mad Men*. Burger Chef was one of the clients of the program's fictional advertising firm, Sterling Cooper. The production crew took Jim's Burgers in Rialto, California, a former Burger Chef building, and painstakingly brought it back to its former glory inside and out.

Vicki's Lunch Van in Montgomery, Alabama, and Jack's Old Fashion Hamburger House in Fort Lauderdale, Florida, are both located in former Burger Chef buildings. They have one other thing in common; both serve awesome old-school burgers.

Burger Queen/Druther's

Year Founded: *1956*

City Founded: *Winter Haven, Florida*

Type: *Regional*

Founders: *Harold and Helen Kite* (Burger Queen); *Tom Hensley* and *Bob Gatewood* (Druther's)

Number of Locations at the Chain's Peak: *217*

Locations Still in Operation: *1*

Signature Burgers: *Queen Burger, Royal Burger, Imperial Burger, Huckleburger,* and *Deluxe Quarter*

Mascots: *Queenie Bee* (1970s) and *Andy Dandytale* (1980s)

Slogans: *"Something Big's Cooking at Burger Queen," "Let's all follow Queenie Bee, it's Burger Queen for me!"* and *"I'd Ruther Go to Druther's Restaurant!"*

In 1956, Harold and Helen Kite opened the first Burger Queen restaurant in Winter Haven, Florida. Outside was a twenty-foot-tall sign featuring a curvaceous woman wearing a crown with wand in hand. "Burger Queen Shake 'n' Burger," "Thick Shakes," "19-cent Broiled Burgers," and "Broasted Chicken 79 cents" were in bold lettering. Tampa neon craftsman John F. Cinchett created the eye-catching sign.

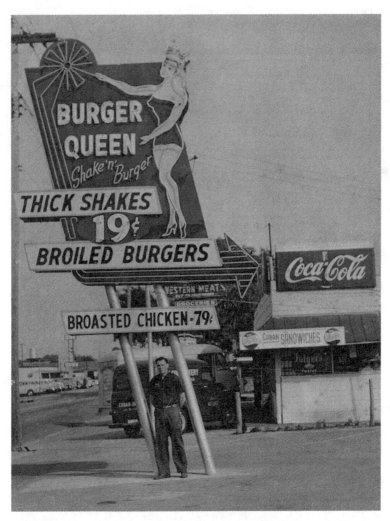

Neon sign maker John F. Cinchett and the Burger Queen
sign he created.

George Clark and Michael Gannon, who were in the Air National Guard together, wanted to enter the fast-food business that was taking the United States by storm. They had attempted to open Dairy Queen, Henry's Hamburgers and McDonald's franchises, but had been turned down for lack of funds. Gannon, who worked in the Taylor Freezer business, met

Harold Kite in Florida and found out about his small but burgeoning Burger Queen chain.

In 1961, Clark and Gannon bought a Burger Queen franchise for five thousand dollars. It took almost another year to convince a bank to lend them the money for the build-out. Their first location, in Middleton, Kentucky, opened on September 23, 1963. At that point, McDonald's was still selling out of a takeout window, while at a Burger Queen restaurant, you could enjoy your meal in the dining room. It was a success from the get-go. Ten years later, fifty Burger Queens were spread across Kentucky, Indiana, and Tennessee.

In March, 1970, American Dairy Queen Inc. of Minneapolis, a.k.a. Dairy Queen, brought a lawsuit against Burger Queen for their use of "Queen" in advertising. DQ claimed that BQ was infringing on fourteen different registered trademarks they owned. As part of the claim, Dairy Queen not only asked for monetary damages but wanted all advertising using "Queen" destroyed. This turn of events was interesting, considering what would happen in 1990.

Burger King purchased the Florida trademark for Burger Queen in 1966. This prevented Harold Kite from expanding in Florida for the next decade, until he bought the trademark in 1976. By that time, George Clark's Burger Queen of Louisville (Gannon having left the company in 1970) had expanded to well over a hundred locations and had become the dominant part of the company. Clark even branched out to a short-lived seafood concept named King Neptune's Seafood Galley in May 1976.

The next few years saw the international expansion of Burger Queen into Canada, Kuwait, Taiwan, the United Arab Emirates, and the United Kingdom. In the UK, they rebranded the business as Huckleberry's. Burger Queen didn't want to offend the Queen of England.

Near the end of March, 1980, a decision was reached to rename the company and its stores. In November, the Burger Queen restaurants in Fulton, Kentucky, and Union, Tennessee, were the first to convert to the new name of Druther's.

A New York consulting firm, Lippincott and Margulies Inc., had suggested the name change from Burger Queen to Druther's and designed the logo. Lippincott and Margulies were also the ones who had told Humble Oil Company to change its name to Exxon, and that had worked out pretty well for them.

The main thought behind the name change was that they were not solely a burger joint, something that seemed lost on many people. All stores officially changed their names in June, 1981. Druther's now had 180 restaurants in five states (Indiana, Kentucky, Ohio, Tennessee, and West Virginia), as well as the franchise rights to the entire world, except for Florida and Georgia.

The company was acquired entirely by Tom Hensley and Bob Gatewood in September 1982. All of the Burger Queen restaurants in Florida were closing their doors by then and never made the conversion to Druther's.

All seventeen of the Huckleberry's locations in the United Kingdom were sold to Grand Metropolitan in 1984; Grand Metropolitan converted them to Wimpy. Ironically enough, Wimpy was known initially as Wimpy Grills. It was founded in Bloomington, Indiana, back in 1934 and crossed the pond in 1954. Shortly after the passing of Wimpy Grills founder Edward Gold in 1977, all of the United States locations closed.

Druther's signed an agreement to become the territory operator for Dairy Queen in September 1990. Just before this, all of the Burger Queen locations in the UAE and Kuwait closed.

One hundred Druther's locations were converted to Dairy Queen by July 1991. This left only the twenty restaurants owned by the company and another fourteen franchises to turn. Many of the restaurants that never switched to Dairy Queen continued to operate as Druther's. They all eventually closed their doors over the next twenty-four years.

Druther's International lives on as Bob Gatewood and Druther's Systems. They co-own eight Dairy Queen restaurants in Indiana, Kentucky, and West Virginia, and are the landlords to another dozen DQs in the region.

There is one independent Druther's Restaurant still fighting the good fight in Campbellsville, Kentucky. Steve McCarty, a second-generation owner-operator, runs what was initially Burger Queen number eighteen. I've been there and met Steve, and I can tell you that it was a highly enjoyable experience to eat at his restaurant.

Carl's Jr.

Year Founded: *1941*
City Founded: *Los Angeles, California*
Type: *Regional*
Founders: *Carl* and *Margaret Karcher*
Number of Locations: *currently at 1,490*
Signature Burger: *Famous Star*
Slogan: *"You've got taste!"*

The Carl's Jr. story began on July 17, 1941, in Los Angeles, California, with a hot dog cart. Carl Karcher was working for Armstrong Bakery in Manhattan Beach, California. He started off wrapping bread, but through hard work was promoted to delivery. While doing deliveries in Los Angeles, he came across a hot dog pushcart with a red umbrella for sale on the corner of Florence and Central.

Lou Richmond, who owned the stand, sold hot dogs, tamales, and drinks. It was for sale for $326. At that moment, Carl didn't have the funds to take him up on the offer, and his wife Margaret didn't like the idea of them going into debt to buy the cart. Back then, it wasn't a practical idea, since they were only a few years removed from the Great Depression.

But Carl was driven. He went to Bank of America to secure a loan for $311 against his 1941 Plymouth. Funny enough, the other fifteen dollars came straight out of Margaret's purse.

The cart the Karchers had bought was known as Hugo's. The Goodyear Blimp used a field near them, so Carl renamed it "The Blimp." Sales for the first day of operation totaled $14.75, which was pretty good, considering they were selling ten-cent hot dogs, chili dogs, and tamales, with drinks at five cents.

Carl kept driving the bakery truck full-time and worked at The Blimp when he was off. Along with some hired help, Margaret worked the stand the rest of its operating hours.

The cart did such brisk business that in May of 1942 a second one followed, then a third in December, and their final cart in early 1943. This was all happening in the middle of World War II, when rations were in full effect and rings of baloney would be substituted for hot dogs.

Carl introduced hamburgers at his fourth cart. He used an ice cream scooper to portion out the burgers before cooking. His first burger was called the 49er, one-third of a pound of beef which sold for 49 cents. There was also a Texas Burger, and a Burger Steak on a Bun, too. The addition of the burgers to their menu was a hit.

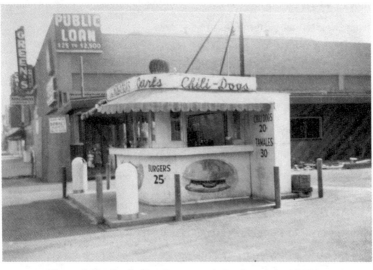

One of the Carl's Hot Dog stands in the early 1940s.

By December, 1943, Carl was comfortable enough with his four carts to quit the bread route. The Karchers had been longing to return to Anaheim, California, and when the opportunity presented itself, they changed gears and opened a full-service restaurant. On January 16, 1945, Carl's Drive-In Barbecue opened up for business. The thirty-seat establishment also had enough parking to accommodate thirty cars. Margaret waited on tables, and Carl cooked up the grub. On the first day, they took in a very respectable $77.64. When hamburgers were added to the menu in 1946, six burgers could fit at a time on the small fifteen-inch grills.

But trouble loomed for the Karchers. The owners of the restaurant property didn't renew the lease and planned to open their own restaurant in the same space. The Karchers were given thirty days to leave the premises.

Carl had to think quick. He ended up buying a garage on property owned by his father-in-law. After four weeks of revamping their new space, they moved into it on the thirtieth day. All of the equipment and furnishings from the original spot made it to the new restaurant.

In 1956, rather than open more of the larger concept Carl's Drive-In Barbecues, Carl opened two Carl's Jrs. in Anaheim and Brea, which were only a hop and a skip away from each other. These smaller restaurants were takeout only. After ordering at the window, you could then sit down at one of the picnic tables under an awning and enjoy your food. This was also the year that the company officially became known as Carl's Jr.

At the close of the 1950s, there were four Carl's Jr. restaurants. Carl's younger brother Donald F. Karcher was then running them and became president in a few years. When the company incorporated as Carl Karcher Enterprises in 1966, they were up to twenty-four locations in Southern California.

The company would try many new concepts over the next years, but none of them had any legs. There were the railroad-themed Carl's Whistle Stop and Scot's Family Restaurants in the mid-1960s; the Sunshine Broiler in the late '70s and early '80s; and probably the best known of these test concepts was Taco de Carlos. This Mexican-themed restaurant appeared in the early 1970s and reached a peak of seventeen locations in early 1979. Between March and April of 1982, eleven Taco de Carlos spots were sold to Del Taco, two to Naugles, and two to Taco Bell.

In the late 1960s, the Happy Star, as he is now known, became the company mascot. Early 1970s ads referred to the star with a face and shoes as "Starman."

In 1975, the company expanded to Northern California after passing the hundred locations mark. Four years later, they opened their first out of state restaurant in Las Vegas, Nevada.

Carl Karcher Enterprises, or CKE, went public in October 1981 with 1.45 million shares of stock offered at $13.50 a share. The money raised was used to expand the number of restaurants, which in 1981 totaled three hundred.

Carl's Jr. had come a long way since their original hot dog cart at this point. The addition of franchising and a menu expansion in 1984 helped them to grow to 534 locations by the end of the decade.

In 1997, Carl's Jr. purchased Hardee's to add to their lineup of restaurants. Today, Carl's Jr. can be mostly found on the West Coast, while Hardee's is mainly on the East Coast. Carl's Jr. and Hardee's currently have over 3,800 locations in forty-four states and forty foreign countries.

Carrols

Year Founded: *1959*
City Founded: *Wood River, Illinois*
Type: *Regional*
Founders: *Leo Moranz* and *Harry Axene*
Number of Locations at the Chain's Peak: *more than 120*
Locations Still in Operation: *None*
Signature Burger: *Club Burger*
Slogan: *"A Serving a Second"*

Carrols originated from the soft-serve ice cream chain Tastee Freez and was named after cofounder Leo Maranz's daughter Carol. Its first location opened in Wood River, Illinois, on July 8, 1959. Carrols was set up as a franchisable concept from the get-go.

Carrols Drive-in System
Opens in WOOD RIVER
648 Wood River Ave., Wood River, Ill.

Across from the Swimming Pool

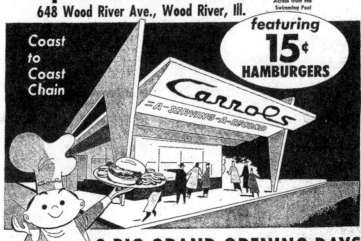

Coast to Coast Chain

featuring 15¢ HAMBURGERS

3 BIG GRAND OPENING DAYS
THURS., FRI., SAT. --- JULY 9, 10, 11

MENU
HAMBURGERS 15¢

Cheeseburgers . . . 19¢
Large 16 oz. Shakes . 20¢
French Fries . . . . . 10¢
Coca Cola . . . 10 & 15¢
Coffee . . . . 10¢
Milk . . . . . . 10¢
Soft Drinks . . 10 & 15¢

FREE!
ORANGE Crush & Root Beer
FREE GIFTS and SOUVENIRS

OPEN FROM 11 A.M. to MIDNIGHT
ALL MEAT Used in Our Hamburgers
100% PURE BEEF!

FREE!
Hamburger
Buy one Get one FREE
on GRAND OPENING DAYS ONLY
2 for 1
LIMIT 4 to a Customer

648 WOOD RIVER AVE. . . . WOOD RIVER, ILL.

Grand Opening ad for Carrol's from the *Alton Evening Telegraph* on July 8, 1959.

Herb Slotnick, who had initially been interested in opening a McDonald's, ended up buying the franchise rights for the New York area. He opened his first Carrols in Syracuse, New York, on June 23, 1960. When the Carrols corporation faced financial difficulties later on, Slotnick took control of the entire chain.

Carrols did very well until McDonald's and Burger King moved into their neck of the woods. These powerhouses outmatched Carrols on advertising and spending wherever necessary. Slotnick saw the handwriting on the wall and made a sound business decision. In 1975, he entered into an agreement with the Burger King Corporation to convert Carrols' locations into BKs over a five-year period.

Starting in 1975, Carrols opened locations in Finland, Sweden, Estonia, Latvia, and Russia. The last existing locations overseas were in Helsinki, Finland. Hesburger, a Finnish restaurant company, bought them out in 2002. The Club Burger was available for a while on the Hesburger menu.

All these years later, ironically enough, Carrols is now the largest franchisee of Burger King, with over eight hundred locations. It is also traded on the New York Stock Exchange under "TAST."

Hamburger Handout

Year Founded: *1952*
City Founded: *Culver City, California*
Type: *Hyper-Local*
Founder: *James Collins*
Number of Locations at the Chain's Peak: *4*
Locations Still in Operation: *None*

Hamburger Handout was a micro burger chain whose founder went on to be a mover and shaker in the expanding food franchise space. In 1952, James Collins' father-in-law owned a corner property with a 110-space trailer park and an eighteen-pump gas station in Culver City, California. There was also an empty building that he wanted Collins to convert into a coffee shop. It made sense with all the folks living in the trailer park and others stopping in to get their vehicle filled.

Once he was mid-remodel, the gentleman from the electrical company, with whom Collins was friendly, asked if he had some free time. They drove two and a half hours away to the original McDonald's in San Bernardino. Collins watched them absolutely kill it for lunch.

Twenty-four hours later, he was back—this time with his father-in-law in tow. They met the McDonald brothers, who showed them around and explained what they were doing, as they did for many others.

Collins didn't waste a minute. He went back to their equipment supplier and asked them to design a hamburger stand. On September 28, 1952, Hamburger Handout opened up shop in Culver City, California. They were busy the moment they opened. The first year alone they did $421,000 in sales with a fifty-one-cent check average. You're talking roughly 800,000 customers buying nineteen-cent hamburgers in just twelve months.

Collins wanted to open more locations, but his father-in-law was not keen on the idea. He believed Collins should be content with their one successful restaurant. So when his in-laws took a trip to Europe in 1957, he bought and fixed up another burger stand, which became Hamburger Handout number two.

Shortly after that, in 1958, they opened a third location. In 1959, they built a brand-new spot from scratch for their fourth Hamburger Handout.

In 1960, Collins visited the owner of the four Burke's Drive-Ins located in San Francisco. Mrs. Burke suggested that he add Kentucky Fried Chicken to the Hamburger Handout menu. Collins considered himself a burger stand purist and didn't like the idea. She insisted they visit Colonel Sanders and wouldn't take no for an answer. She called up a travel agency and bought them two tickets on American Airlines to Louisville, Kentucky.

The Colonel showed up during a snowstorm to pick them up. With chains on his tires, he drove them to his house in Shelbyville, Kentucky, where they spent three days. By the time he left, Collins had signed a franchise agreement for all four Hamburger Handouts.

In 1961, Collins partnered with his UCLA Beta brothers Walt McBee and Rush Backer to open some take home Kentucky Fried Chicken stores in Anaheim, Tustin, and Costa Mesa, California. Collins did such a great job that he became the Southern California Franchise Representative for Kentucky Fried Chicken in 1963. Within five years, he opened up 240 franchisee KFC stores, including twenty-seven of his own between the Mexican border and San Luis Obispo, California.

While Collins was redirecting all of his energies to his KFC gig, Hamburger Handout suffered. McDonald's was also now spreading throughout California with franchises that hurt Hamburger Handout's sales. This neglect ultimately caused the closing of all four Hamburger Handout locations within the next year or so.

Meanwhile...

Del Johnson, who was Hamburger Handout's Minick-Wilshire Dairies ice cream salesman, stopped into Collins' office in 1957. He had an idea for a sizzling steakhouse after reading a story in the Wall Street Journal about the Tad's Steak House chain. The "sizzling" by the way, refers to a steak sizzling when added to a heated metal plate. Tad's locations in

New York City, Chicago, and San Francisco featured a steak, baked potato, and salad combo for $1.09. Johnson's only problem was that he didn't have a cent to his name.

Collins' father-in-law offered Johnson a small trailer by the gas station to help his dream become a reality. He also signed a bank note for Johnson to the tune of twenty thousand dollars. Collins lent him a fifteen-pound fryer and a five-foot grill. They bought some light fixtures, redwood tables, and chairs to fill the space.

On January 27, 1958, Del's Sizzler Steak House opened with thirty-two seats inside and about another thirty-two outside on the patio under some umbrellas. At Sizzler, as it would later be known, you would place your order at the counter and receive a number. When your number was called, you would pick up your food. The simple menu consisted of three different steaks, a steak sandwich, a hamburger, and fried shrimp. Their quick-service operation allowed them to sell as many as two hundred quarter-pound hamburgers a day.

By July, 1967, Johnson owned four restaurants and had franchised 160 Sizzler restaurants. He was ready to retire and asked Collins if he'd be interested in purchasing the company from him. Collins, along with McBee and Backer, bought the Sizzler company for $985,000.

The trio then hit the road and visited every location. Thirty-five of the restaurants that were struggling to make ends meet were broken off from the company and changed their name. Now that they had cut some of the company fat, they would consolidate all of their businesses.

In the summer of 1968, Collins combined the Sizzler chain, his twenty-seven Kentucky Fried Chickens, the locations with his two UCLA friends, and a small two truck wholesale company to create Collins Food International Inc.

On November 15, 1968, Sizzler went public with three hundred thousand shares at eighteen dollars each. It netted the new company five million dollars, which was used to develop the Sizzler chain. It was then that they started to make menu changes to move Sizzler away from its fast-food beginnings.

Hardee's

Year Founded: *1960*
City Founded: *Greenville, North Carolina*
Type: *Regional*
Founder: *Wilber Hardee*
Number of Locations: *currently well over 2,000*
Signature Burgers: *Huskee, Big Twin,* and
 Big Deluxe
Slogan: *"We're out to win you over."*

On an empty lot in Greenville, North Carolina, Wilber Hardee (not Wilbur as it is commonly misspelled) opened his first namesake restaurant on September 3, 1960. He had visited the first McDonald's in North Carolina and watched as it grossed $168 over one hour during lunchtime. Wilber was convinced that he could recreate what they were doing and do it better. He took a picture of the restaurant and drove home to plan out what would become Hardee's.

Wilber found someone to build him a small building in a similar style to a McDonald's, using red and white tiles similar to those that covered the iconic McDonald's structures. The first Hardee's didn't have a dining room, tables, a drive-thru, or even carhops. What it did have was two windows, one for ordering and another for picking up food.

The first Hardee's menu featured fifteen-cent hamburgers, twenty-cent cheeseburgers, fries, fried apple pies, milkshakes, and soft drinks. McDonald's was cooking their burgers on a flat-top, while Hardee's used chargrills, which he believed would give him the edge over the golden arches.

Less than a year after the McDonald's location that had inspired him had set up shop in Greensboro, North Carolina, Hardee's opened its doors. The public loved it, and the long lines at the windows proved it.

Wilber started on plans to open the second location a year later in Rocky Mount, North Carolina. It was here that the trajectory of the Hardee's chain would change forever. He met accountant Leonard Rawls and his friend James Gardner. The duo convinced Wilber that by selling Hardee's franchises, they could all be set up financially for life. Hardee's Drive-Ins would be incorporated following their agreement, which oddly enough had no money changing hands.

On May 7, 1961, the second Hardee's opened up in Rocky Mount under their new corporation. It was another successful location for them. But things were not good between the partners.

Wilber has given different versions of what happened next. The best known was that he lost a poker game against Rawls and Gardner, and along with that, the controlling interest in Hardee's. In another story, they got him drunk and had him sign away any control of future franchise sales. Whatever happened, the result was that all three men had an equal say in the new corporation, which left Wilber outvoted in the company he had founded. He was extremely angry with the situation; he had signed away everything for twenty or thirty-seven thousand dollars, depending on who was telling the story. When he signed Hardee's away, there were five stores total.

By August 1961, Rawls had become president of Hardee's with Gardner as vice president. The first Hardee's franchisees were their friends and acquaintances. In mid-August 1963, Hardee's Food Systems went public, selling four-dollar shares that provided three hundred thousand dollars to develop more restaurants. In 1966, James Gardner stepped down as vice president of the company when he was elected to the U.S. House of Representatives.

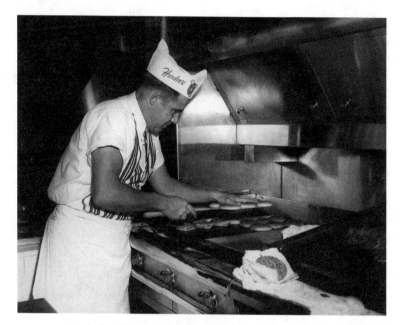

Hardee's grill man taking care of business in the early 1960s.

Between the late 1960s and early 1980s, Hardee's expanded, opening hundreds of new restaurants and purchasing other burger chains and converting them to the Hardee's brand.

One of those was Sandy's, which was originally going to be run as its own separate company. They didn't even cook burgers the same way. At least that was the plan in late November 1971, when the acquisition of the 207-location chain occurred. But by 1973, the plan had changed, and now 90 percent of Sandy's would become Hardee's. The other 10 percent would undergo name changes and then operate independently.

In February 1981, Hardee's merged with Imasco Ltd. of Montreal, Canada, and became a subsidiary under their banner. On March 10, 1982, Imasco purchased Burger Chef for forty-four million dollars. The conversion from Burger Chef to Hardee's was gradual, giving the franchises the opportunity to stay on board or go their separate ways.

Hardee's also purchased the Utah-based twenty-eight location burger chain Dee's Drive-Ins in August of 1982. This Dee's is not to be confused with the Dee's Drive Inn still open in Louisa, Kentucky, which is a great old-school spot with curb service. By the end of 1982, Hardee's was at over 2,150 locations in thirty-eight states.

Of course, it didn't end there. Hardee's purchased the Roy Rogers Roast Beef and Fried Chicken chain in April 1990, putting Hardee's at almost four thousand restaurants.

Then, in a weird turn of events, after a rough 1996, during which Hardee's lost ten million dollars, the company was bought by the 675-unit Carl's Jr. for $327 million. It appeared that the plan was to convert all Hardee's into Carl's Jr. restaurants, but that never materialized.

The charbroiled burgers from Carl's Jr. replaced Hardee's current crop of sandwiches. The popular Hardee's breakfast was added to all Carl's Jr. locations. The Carl's Jr. Happy Star mascot would now be a part of the Hardee's logo.

Today, Carl's Jr. is predominantly found on the West Coast while Hardee's is on the East Coast of the United States. Hardee's and Carl's Jr. now have over 3,800 locations in forty-four states and forty foreign countries.

Henry's Hamburgers

Year Founded: *1954*
City Founded: *Chicago, Illinois*
Type: *National*
Founder: *Bresler's Ice Cream Company*
Number of Locations at the Chain's Peak: *200*
Locations Still in Operation: *None*
Signature Burger: *Big Henry*
Slogans: *"Aren't you hungry for a Henry's?"* and *"Head for Henry's"*

In 1954, Henry's Hamburgers was born when Bresler's Ice Cream Company caught the fast-food fever that was taking over the United States. Their new burger concept was perfect for selling more of their ice cream in malts and milkshakes, as well as expanding the reach of their brand. The name "Henry" was a tribute to Henry Bresler, one of the founders of Bresler's Ice Cream Company.

The inspiration for Henry's Hamburgers was Culver City's Hamburger Handout and San Bernardino's McDonald's. The first store was in Chicago, Illinois, and six years later, there were twenty-one restaurants in that area alone. Funny enough, the kitchen designer for Henry's prototype location ended up joining McDonald's design team.

On April 26, 1960, Henry's Drive-In, as they were legally known, went public with one hundred thousand shares of stock at $2.50. By then, there were one hundred Henry's Hamburgers locations either open or in different stages of construction.

Henry's peaked at around two hundred locations in the late 1960s. In December, 1974, the corporate name was changed to Amfood Industries, Inc. But a lack of drive-thrus and money for national advertising took its toll on Henry's, and restaurants were now closing at an alarming rate.

In May, 1981, they were down to ten Henry's locations. Amfood Industries filed for bankruptcy in October of 1985. They had lost $750,000 on sales of $7.9 million, it was the final blow that did in Henry's Hamburgers.

If you're still looking for a Henry's Hamburger fix, you're in luck! The Benton Harbor, Michigan, location, which opened in April, 1959, is still open for business. We have to thank current owner Dave Slavicek for keeping this burger landmark alive.

In-N-Out

Year Founded: *1948*
City Founded: *Baldwin Park, California*
Type: *Regional*
Founders: *Harry Snyder* and *Esther Snyder*
Number of Locations: *currently over 335*
Signature Burger: *Double-Double*
Slogan: *"Quality you can taste, Cleanliness you can see"*

On October 22, 1948, In-N-Out debuted in Baldwin Park, California. Fifty-seven burgers were sold on that opening day. Little did Harry and Esther Snyder know that their drive-thru hamburger stand would create a rabid following that exists to this day.

The very first In-N-Out was on the southwest corner of what is now Interstate 10 and Francisquito Avenue. A crucial element to its success was the two-way speaker box that allowed drivers to place their orders. There was no indoor seating, and there were no carhops.

The original In-N-Outs were double drive-thrus. The kitchen was located in the building that serviced the cars. Because of their size, food and supplies were kept in a separate building just across from the drive-thru. There was an awning for the few tables provided along with a walk-up service window.

In-N-Out placed their locations near new roads, an excellent fit for California Hot Rod culture.

The original menu featured twenty-five-cent hamburgers, thirty-cent cheeseburgers, fifteen-cent fries, and ten-cent bottled soda pop. The drinks were 7-UP, Coke, cream soda, Delaware Punch, orange, root beer, Pepsi, and strawberry. Cigarettes were sold, too, but didn't last long. Milkshakes weren't officially added to the menu until 1975.

When eating in your car, things can get messy, so at In-N-Out, you'd be offered a lap mat, a.k.a. a placemat. Back in the day, Harry would make custom lap mats out of the brown wax paper that housed the buns. He later switched to pink butcher paper. These days, they're all branded with In-N-Out information.

The In-N-Out secret menu (which has not been secret since the Internet age) features the "Animal Style" burger. Customer demand in 1961 spawned the mustard-cooked beef burger with lettuce, tomato, pickle, and extra spread with grilled onions on a burger bun.

A few years later, In-N-Out hung a banner in the store asking customers to "Try a Double-Double," their double cheese double burger patty. Its popularity would make it a permanent addition to their menu.

Harry Snyder was a big fan of the film *It's a Mad, Mad, Mad, Mad World*; its plot had its characters searching for a hidden treasure that was under "the big W" made by four palm trees. In 1972, the first pair of crossed palm trees were planted at an In-N-Out forming an "X." It's a tradition that continues to this day.

Rich Snyder became president of In-N-Out at the age of twenty-four when his father Harry passed away in 1976; at the time, there were eighteen locations. Over the next seventeen years, this would grow rapidly (though not fast enough for their fan base) to ninety-three.

Their twenty-first location opened in 1979 in Ontario, California, with a few innovations. It was the first In-N-Out with a dining room and only a single drive-thru.

It wasn't until 1990 that In-N-Out opened their first location outside of Los Angeles. The San Diego area In-N-Out was their fifty-seventh restaurant. Just two years later, in 1992, they opened up in Las Vegas, Nevada.

On December 15, 1993, Rich Snyder died in a tragic plane crash shortly after the opening of In-N-Out's ninety-third restaurant in Fresno, California. His brother Guy Snyder, who succeeded him as president, continued to expand In-N-Out to 140 locations until his untimely death in 1999.

Esther Snyder took the reins of the company she had founded with her husband. Their continued expansion brought them into Arizona in 2000.

After Esther's passing in 2006, Mark Taylor, vice president of operations, took the helm. Under his tutelage, In-N-Outs sprouted up in Utah.

In 2010, Lynsi Snyder, the daughter of Guy and only grandchild of Esther and Harry, became In-N-Out's sixth company president. She owned the company through a trust after Esther passed away and received full control of In-N-Out on her thirty-fifth birthday in May 2017.

Lynsi expanded In-N-Out into Texas in 2011 and Oregon in 2015 and plans to move into Colorado and possibly New Mexico. All new restaurants must be within a day's drive of the nearest commissary where the fresh never frozen burgers are produced.

There's something unique about the culture the Snyders have built with In-N-Out that would change if they ever went public or sold the company. Rich Snyder told Forbes in 1989:

> *"My feeling is that I would be prostituting what my parents made by doing that. There is money to be made by doing those things, but you lose something, and I don't want to lose what I was raised with all my life."*

You gotta love that.

In-N-Out Quirky Facts

Up until 2005, you could walk into any In-N-Out and order as many burgers and slices of cheese you wanted in your sandwich. There was an additional cost per patty and slice, but no limit to your meat imagination.

On October 31, 2004, blogger Will Young walked into an In-N-Out in Las Vegas and ordered a Double-Double with ninety-eight extra patties and cheese. He was charged $97.66 for the 100 x 100 (100 burger patties, 100 slices of cheese). He and his seven friends actually ate the entire thing.

Once the picture started making the rounds on the Internet, In-N-Out management rejected orders of anything larger than a 4 x 4.

Jack in the Box

Founded: *August 1950*
City Founded: *San Diego, California*
Type: *Regional*
Founder: *Robert Oscar Peterson*
Number of Locations: *currently over 2,200*
Signature Burger: *Jumbo Jack*
Slogan: *"The food is better at the Box."*

Before we can jump into Jack in the Box, we need to go back about ten years before it started. In 1941, Robert Oscar Peterson founded a chain of restaurants called Topsy's Drive-In in San Diego, California. A few years later, he renamed those restaurants, as well as the Coronado and National City, California, locations, Oscar's Drive Inn (his middle name). They also underwent a thematic overhaul featuring a circus decor complete with clown drawings.

The rights to an intercom ordering concept that had been pioneered at the Chatterbox in Anchorage, Alaska, were purchased from its founder, George Manos, in 1947.

During August in 1950, the location in San Diego was renamed Jack in the Box. A good part of the restaurant's initial popularity can be attributed to the combination of the intercom ordering and the drive-thru window. Later on, there was a small clown head that sat on the top of a large menu board in the drive-thru with the phrase "Pull forward, Jack will speak to you" on the side.

Some of the Oscar's locations were redesigned and became Jack in the Box. A giant Jack in the Box clown on the buildings could be spotted from a distance as they looked down over their customers.

The Jack in the Box menu has always featured a hamburger. But it's not the most popular item, the taco is. In 2017, there were 554 million tacos sold.

In 1960, Peterson created Foodmaker, Inc. as the parent company for Jack in the Box. Over the next three years, they were busily opening their first eateries outside of California in Arizona and Texas. By 1966, they had hit two hundred company owned eateries.

Foodmaker became a subsidiary of the Ralston Purina Company in 1968. This marked a tremendous growth period for them, with more than a thousand Jack in the Box drive-thrus in the mid-1970s. I can't leave this era without mentioning their popular series of commercials that featured child actor Rodney Allen Rippy in the early 1970s.

But their quick expansion ended up hurting them. To regroup, Jack in the Box sold off 232 locations in the state of Florida and the Chicago, Detroit, and Kansas City markets.

They also rethought their marketing plan. They were looking to go after a more adult and affluent crowd with new menu items and redecorated eating establishments. They unleashed a series of commercials where the Jack in the Box clown was blown up. One memorable commercial featured a little old lady who shouted:

"Waste him!"

To focus on the adult specialty sandwich market, they added a popular Swiss and bacon burger. In 1989, a sourdough burger was added, which would be renamed in 1997. The Sourdough Jack, as it is now known, is my favorite Jack in the Box burger. A burger patty is served up on toasted sourdough bread with tomatoes, Swiss cheese, bacon, ketchup, and mayo.

In early 1982, Jack in the Box finally began to franchise. All the changes made to the menu and decor started to pay dividends financially. Sales had risen to $61.4 million in 1984 from just $36 million only four years earlier.

In January of 1985, the Seattle, Washington, market was the first to test a name change to Monterey Jack's. Employees wore "No more clownin' around" shirts. Eventually, sixty locations would be renamed in Albuquerque, New Mexico; Beaumont, Texas; and St. Louis, Missouri. But the change did very little for them, since most customers still referred to them as Jack in the Box; so the name returned to all of those spots on May 5, 1986.

In the midst of the name change, a group of investors along with some of the management from Foodmaker completed a leveraged buyout of Jack in the Box from Ralston Purina in 1985. They returned the company's focus to its core item, the hamburger, while still adding things like seasoned curly fries.

Nowadays, most folks associate Jack in the Box with their mascot, Jack Box. His head was patterned after the original clown that adorned their old drive-thru boxes. In December 1994, a new advertising campaign positioned him as the fictional founder and CEO of the company. In a nod to his likeness' removal from the company in 1980, the first commercial had Jack retaliating by blowing up Jack in the Box's board of directors.

Jack in the Box Quirky Facts

The return of Jack Box ignited something entirely unintended, a craze for antenna balls. Jack in the Box has either sold or given away more than twenty-eight million antenna balls with Jack's likeness since his return.

Several locations were converted to a new fast-casual concept called JBX Grill in March of 2004. It cut out most of the cheaper items on the Jack in the Box menu and focused on higher quality fare. The modern decor included a fireplace. But the idea was scrapped altogether in September, 2005.

Jack in The Box recently captured the Guinness World Records title for largest coupon in 2015. They created a two thousand-square-foot "Buy One, Get One Free" voucher for the Buttery Jack burger. To actually set the record, the coupon needed to be redeemed. Since it would not fit through the front door of the restaurant, twelve people helped carry it to the drive-thru to complete the transaction.

Red Barn

Year Founded: *1961*
City Founded: *Springfield, Ohio*
Type: *National*
Founders: *James Kirst, Martin A. Levine,* and *Don L. Six*
Number of Locations at the Chain's Peak: *317*
Locations Still in Operation: *None*
Signature Burger: *Big Barney and Barnbuster*
Slogan: *"When the Hungries hit...hit the Red Barn."*

In 1961, Red Barn was founded in Springfield, Ohio, by James Kirst, Martin A. Levine, and Don L. Six. The buildings of the original restaurants were shaped like a barn with high ceilings and large front facing glass window panes. The building design was patented the year after opening, although I can't imagine that someone else would have attempted to copy it. Better safe than sorry, I guess. Later locations had a more standard fast-food type look to them.

When Richard O. Kearns purchased the chain in 1963, the headquarters was moved to Dayton, Ohio, and then in August, 1964, to Fort Lauderdale, Florida. It was an odd move since there were few Red Barns in Florida.

Red Barn was not only known for their burgers. Fried chicken was also another favorite. In July of 1967, they opened a fried chicken spinoff restaurant called Red Barn Chicken Pantry in Kansas City, Missouri, and in September, 1967, added another in Dayton, Ohio. They expanded to a few more states, but by late 1971, all of the locations had closed down.

Three Red Barn mascots were used in commercials, in store advertising, and as promotional giveaways for kids. The main one was Hamburger Hungry, who looked eerily similar to Ernie from Sesame Street with a face like a hamburger bun. Chicken Hungry was a giant chicken leg with eyes, a mouth, a nose, and arms with white gloves on its hands. Big Fish Hungry was a big blue fish with the same attributes as Chicken Hungry. These guys were absolutely frightening. I can't believe Red Barn thought enough of them to produce a set of stuffed animals, which is now a highly sought-after collectible set. For the record, I have a set at my Burger Museum in Miami.

In the late 1960s, Servomation took over Red Barn Systems. But by 1978, Red Barn's days were numbered after Motel 6's parent company purchased them. At that point, the more than three hundred location chain was found in forty-one states. But the new company showed little to no interest in Red Barn and ceased all advertising. Franchise leases were not renewed and were allowed to expire.

In 1983, twenty-six Red Barn stores did not take this lying down. They banded together and rebranded themselves as The Farm with pretty much the same menu items, but under different names. By 1988, Red Barn restaurants were no more. However, there is one last location of The Farm still open in Racine, Wisconsin.

Sandy's

> **Year Founded:** *1956*
> **City Founded:** *Urbana, Illinois*
> **Type:** *Regional*
> **Founders:** *W.K. Davidson, Gus Lundberg, Robert C. Wenger,* and *Paul White*
> **Number of Locations at the Chain's Peak:** *210*
> **Locations Still in Operation:** *None*
> **Signature Burger:** *Big Scott*
> **Slogan:** *"Thrift n Swift"* and *"Come as You Are"*

While traveling from Illinois to a restaurant industry convention in California, friends Paul White and Robert C. Wenger ran into their old Army friend Dick McDonald. Dick and his brother Mac had opened the first McDonald's in San Bernardino, and Ray Kroc was already selling franchise rights. Dick suggested to his friends that they visit Kroc at his Des Plaines location.

Gus Lundberg, known for his leadership skills, was enlisted to join the duo; and along with the well-funded W.K. Davidson and his restaurant experience, he filled out the fourth spot of what was to become a McDonald's franchise.

In December, 1955, after acquiring what they thought were the McDonald's rights to central Illinois, the group was on their way to open one of the few golden arches outside of California at the time. Their first McDonald's opened in June of 1956 near the University of Illinois in Urbana, Illinois. It did well enough that they wanted to open locations in Decatur and Peoria, Illinois, but Kroc informed them those cities were not part of the central Illinois territory.

The partners had already invested in building out the Peoria location. So they decided to open their own restaurant in that location instead after incorporating as Sandy's Inc. in 1957.

On August 8, 1958, Sandy's number one opened in Peoria. It featured a Scottish theme thought to be a shot fired at McDonald's, which had a Scottish family crest on some of their earlier signs. The menu included a fifteen-cent hamburger, a twenty-cent milkshake, and a ten-cent bag of french fries.

McDonald's filed a breach of contract lawsuit against Sandy's, and a seven-year court battle ensued. It ended with an out of court settlement in 1965, which specified that their Urbana location would revert to being a McDonald's.

By 1966, Sandy's had grown to 121 locations in five states. As the end of the 1960s neared, they were in dire need of cash to keep up with the television advertising now being used by their competitors.

Hardee's stepped in to save the day—or so it seemed. After the merger, the new company was 550 locations strong in thirty-four states. After the purchase of Sandy's stock on November 30, 1971, it was thought each company would be run independently.

But somewhere along the line, the plans changed. In 1973, ninety percent of Sandy's locations became Hardee's. The remaining ten percent changed their name to things like Bucky's, Sandie's, and Zandy's so as not to infringe on the Sandy's name. By 1979, the Sandy's name had disappeared altogether.

Wetson's

Year Founded: *1959*
City Founded: *Levittown, New York*
Type: *Regional*
Founders: *Errol and Herbert Wetanson*
Number of Locations at the Chain's Peak: *70*
Locations Still in Operation: *None*
Signature Burger: *The Big W*
Slogans: *"Look for the Orange Circles"* and *"Buy a bagful"*

After visiting a McDonald's, Herb Wetanson was inspired to open a similar restaurant. He and his brother Errol founded Wetson's in 1959.

The first Wetson's opened in Levittown, New York, in a former Mayflower Coffee and Donut Shop space. Their only real competition at that time was White Castle. Wetson's slogans were riffs on McDonald's "Look for the Golden Arches" and White Castle's "Buy 'em by the Sack."

The original restaurants featured a walk-up window with very few outdoor seats and four bright orange circles on the left and right side of the roof. The Wetson's menu featured fifteen-cent hamburgers, fresh cut fries at ten cents, soft drinks, and shakes. It was in line with most fast-food joints of the time. Later on, they added their signature sandwich, the Big W.

Wetson's opened seventy locations in Connecticut and New Jersey, mostly in Brooklyn, Long Island, and Staten Island, New York. They eventually added a couple of mascots to appeal to children: Wetty, a female clown, and Sonny, a male clown.

In the early 1970s, Burger King and McDonald's entered their market, and Wetson's began to struggle against these national chains. Shortly after Wetson's filed for bankruptcy, the New York Times announced on March 4, 1975, that Nathan's would be merging with the remaining twenty-eight locations. Once the merger was completed, the Wetson's were converted to the new concept Nathan's Junior's restaurants.

Wetson's was gone, but maybe not forever. In 2016 National Food Brands Marketing Inc. purchased the Wetson's trademark, which means there's hope for a comeback.

Whataburger

Year Founded: *1950*
City Founded: *Corpus Christi, Texas*
Type: *Regional*
Founders: *Paul Burton* and *Harmon Dobson*
Number of Locations: *currently over 824*
Signature Burger: *Whataburger*
Slogan: *"Just like you like it."*

Paul Barton and Harmon Dobson founded Whataburger. They opened their first restaurant in Corpus Christi, Texas, on August 8, 1950, right across from Del Mar College.

Only a couple of months earlier, Dobson had met Burton and decided to finance a small hamburger joint. His goal was to create a better burger that was so large to hold, it would take two hands. The burger also had to taste so good that when you took that first bite, you would exclaim "What a burger!" The "Whataburger" trademark was made official by the office of the Texas Secretary of State on June 23, 1950.

The first Whataburger location was a modest building, but they later became known for their iconic giant A-frame buildings. The roofs were colored with orange and white stripes because Dobson, a pilot, wanted to be able to spot his restaurants from the sky. In 1961, the first of these buildings opened in Odessa, Texas.

Dobson was known to fly over the skies of Corpus Christi with a "Whataburger" banner in tow. His great advertising idea didn't end there. He would also drop a bunch of coupons for free Whataburgers.

Dobson wanted something more massive than the standard two-ounce burger patties on a small bun. His Whataburger was a quarter-pound patty grilled to order with lettuce, three slices of tomato, four pickles, chopped onions, mustard, and ketchup. The larger burger called for a more substantial bun. A five-inch bun did not exist yet. After finding a company that could make the custom pans and molds, they were in business.

On opening day, the menu consisted of twenty-five cent burgers, chips, and drinks. The first day's take was fifty dollars with ninety-one more trickling in over the next couple of days. On the fourth day, Dobson wrote in his diary: "Big day–$141.80–Christ–What a workhorse. 551 burgers." Yup, they were onto something, all right.

The partnership between Burton and Dobson ended in 1951 over a disagreement about raising the price of their burgers from twenty-five to thirty cents. Under their new agreement, Burton owned all franchises in the San Antonio, Texas area. He was a loyal Whataburger operator until he passed away in 1970. Dobson retained control of the rest of the Whataburger company.

Dobson, who had a great sense of humor, posted a giant sign outside the restaurant with this message: "Folks, we priced our burgers too low, and we lost our shirts. Sorry, but we gotta raise the price to thirty cents." Customers found the sign charming and were not about to give up their Whataburger over five cents. Funny enough, a few short months later he raised the price again to thirty-five cents.

In 1953 the first Whataburger franchise was sold to Joe Andrews. The first Whataburger restaurant outside of Texas opened in Pensacola, Florida in 1959. Eight years later, they had almost forty locations and were in Arizona, Florida, Tennessee, and Texas.

On April 11, 1967, tragedy struck. Dobson took off in his Cessna Skymaster airplane and something went wrong after takeoff. The aircraft crashed, killing him and his passenger instantly. Dobson's will stated his desire for Whataburger to continue after his death, and his wife Grace followed in his footsteps and led the company. Their son Tom Dobson was later elected president of Whataburger in December 1993.

The eighties were not a good decade for Whataburger. They lost focus on their signature dish, the Whataburger. Tom, along with his new management team, turned around the company's fortunes. They revitalized their relationships with the franchisees, improved their marketing efforts, and made sure their locations received a facelift. Whataburger was proclaimed a Texas Treasure during the Seventy-seventh Session of the Texas Legislature in 2001.

Just as Harmon Dobson asked in his will, Whataburger has stood the test of time and continues to be a business that is family owned and operated, by his children Hugh, Lynne, and Tom.

Chapter

9

A BETTER BURGER REVIVAL

It's easy to get caught up in the fast food world of burgers, and for some folks, that's all they've ever known. As a child, I was gradually introduced to a world where a "better burger" existed. My food blog *Burger Beast* was founded during the early beginnings of the rebirth of the burger in 2008 and 2009. During the intervening years between the Burger Wars, the price battles (including the dollar menu), and the declining quality of the burger, some restaurants were fighting the good fight quietly in the background.

When I was a kid, I distinctly remember eating at Tony Roma's. My entire family ordered ribs, since it was the thing to get there. I was not having any of that jazz, so I, of course, went for old faithful, a.k.a. whatever burger was on the restaurant's menu. I was served a bigger burger than I had ever seen, smothered in BBQ sauce and topped with melted cheese. I didn't know what to make of it. I had never seen a burger from a restaurant that was not Burger King or McDonald's. I was hooked, and when my dad would grill at home, I would drown, not cover, the beef patty in BBQ sauce. Now that I think of it, my version was really gross.

Fuddruckers

Fuddruckers became my next obsession when they opened up in Miami's Pinecrest neighborhood in March 1984. I enjoyed the whole vibe of the place. While waiting in line to place your order, you could see into their "meat shop," with hanging carcasses and a butcher cutting up the soon-to-be burgers. After being called up to the counter to pick up your order, there was a giant salad-type bar filled with fresh chopped onions, tomatoes, lettuce, and much more—the list went on and on.

It was right across from their honey mustard, which went perfectly with their skin-on fries. The honey mustard also sticks out in my memory, since my mom wouldn't allow me to order cheese for my burger due to an allergy I had at the time. I was forced to secretly use their nacho cheese cauldron, right next to the golden honey mustard sauce, to squirt out some of the neon orange stuff onto my bottom bun. On the way out, there was also a bakery to get desserts after your meal, which was also where the buttery buns for the burgers were baked.

Culver's

During the mid-1980s, Fuddruckers was rapidly expanding across the US, but if you were in Sauk City, Wisconsin, then you might have been lucky enough to see the opening of the first Culver's on July 18, 1984. For almost ten years, you could only get Culver's ButterBurgers and Frozen Custard in Wisconsin. They expanded slowly to twenty-five states over the following thirty-five years.

The first time I heard about Culver's was from my late friend Spencer Block. He was from Wisconsin and mentioned them pretty much every time we spoke. He wanted me to go to a Milwaukee Brewers game with him and then hit up Culver's afterward, but it never came to pass. When Culver's finally opened in Florida, I made the almost two-hour trek to Naples with my cousin Fred. We were not disappointed.

Five Guys

Five Guys Burgers and Fries was founded in 1986 by Janie and Jerry Murrell and their four sons. Eventually, a fifth son was born, and he replaced dad as the fifth guy. The company was opening locations at a gradual pace until franchising began in 2003. That's why Five Guys seemed like an overnight success story to some, since one minute they weren't here and the next they were.

Another reason for the interest in Five Guys was the simplicity of the menu. Many burger joints' menus were too bloated, so Five Guys took it back in an old-school direction with an uncomplicated menu of burgers, hot dogs, and fresh cut fries. Their great tasting food explains why there are now more than 1,500 Five Guys Burgers and Fries locations worldwide.

Johnny Rockets

Johnny Rockets debuted with twenty stools in an 840 square foot space in Los Angeles, California, on June 6, 1986. Eventually, the new Johnny Rockets locations added tables and booths in larger areas to accommodate them. Founder Ronn Teitelbaum said the decor was inspired by The Incline, a diner from his youth in 1940s Santa Monica, California. The paper-jacketed hamburgers, counter seating, and minimalist menu of burgers, fries, shakes, flavored colas, and apple pie came from the Apple Pan in Los Angeles.

I never ate at Johnny Rockets when it first popped up in Miami. My friends would talk to me about it, but I steered clear of going to the mall where one was located unless there was the added incentive of an arcade. My first real meal at Johnny Rockets was on a Royal Caribbean cruise ship. The booth type seating was on an outdoor deck facing the ocean with a calming breeze. It made for ideal weather to sit and enjoy burgers, fries, and shakes.

Red Robin

Red Robin may have been founded in September, 1969, but its name didn't gain prominence until commercials aired nationwide with that catchy jingle, "Red Robin YUM!" around 2007. The closest Red Robin to me was in Fort Myers, Florida, over two hours away.

Red Robin serves larger burgers, or as they like to refer to them, gourmet burgers. It's a full-service restaurant with an array of appetizers, preselected burger combinations, and a full bar of libations. I'm a steak fry kind of guy, so I love their bottomless steak fries deal with the purchase of a burger.

Fatburger

Many of its contemporaries cut corners by switching to frozen beef patties and using heat lamps to keep their sandwiches warm, but Fatburger never did. In 1947, Lovie Yancey founded Fatburger as Mr. Fatburger in Los Angeles. I was lucky enough to eat at Fatburger for the first time on their home turf when visiting my late grandmother in Glendale, California. Then when I was old enough to gamble, I'd go to Las Vegas and a grab a Fatburger on the strip.

Later on, Queen Latifah franchised a couple of locations in South Florida, including one that was four spots over from the Metro PCS cell phone store I managed in Coral Gables. I loved watching them place the fresh beef patty on the flat-top and then add cheese and mustard to round out a tasty burger specimen.

Speaking of Queen Latifah, a bunch of rappers, like the Beastie Boys, Ice Cube, Notorious BIG, and Tupac, have shown Fatburger some love in their songs.

Habit Burger

Another chain from California is The Habit Burger Grill, founded on November 15, 1969, in Santa Barbara. Over the last few years, they've been spreading their wings around the US. They were family owned until 2007, when the private equity firm that purchased them began franchising and then a few years later took the company public.

Currently located in over ten states with the majority of their locations in California, they expanded to Miami a few years ago with their fresh beef charbroiled burgers. The Charburgers really do taste like a burger cooked up in your backyard, but the best part is no mess or clean up.

Freddy's Frozen Custard

Freddy's Frozen Custard & Steakburgers have only been around since 2002, but this Wichita, Kansas, chain is one to keep an eye on. I love that they hail from the same town where White Castle first opened its doors.

My family and I were driving around Orlando, Florida, when we came across a brightly lit, brand spanking new burger restaurant calling us to visit. Once inside, my first thought was that the look of Freddie's was very reminiscent of Steak 'n Shake.

Their thin griddled burgers were near perfection and served up with pickles, mustard, and onion. You will need to eat a double to really grasp the taste. Please keep all of that garden stuff out of this.

Smashburger

By the time Smashburger was founded by Tom Ryan in 2007, he had already made quite a name for himself in the restaurant industry. He was the creator of Pizza Hut's Stuffed Crust Pizza and the infamous McGriddle sandwich from McDonald's.

The name Smashburger comes from the cooking technique of smashing the beef on the griddle, which creates a beautiful meat crust on it. This is my favorite style of burger, and Smashburger does it right. I always order the double with cheese, mustard, onion, and pickles.

One of the most stressful things I've ever been asked to do was being Smashburger's celebrity smasher when they were inaugurating their first restaurant in South Florida. I've cooked thousands of burgers in my lifetime using a variety of techniques, but never with all eyes and cameras focused on me. I was nervous, but did a pretty good job, I think. Google "Smashburger celebrity smasher," and you can watch the video on YouTube.

Shake Shack

Miami wasn't exactly a hotbed of burger activity until Shake Shack announced the opening of a South Beach Shake Shack location with the tagline "MIAMI has a new VICE" in neon green. It was November 2009, and a good two and a half years after their people's choice win at the Super Bowl of burger competitions, the South Beach Wine & Food Festival Burger Bash.

Shake Shack had made a name for itself online with foodies. They had taken the burger concept to its most primordial state, with great simple ingredients all dressed up in a neon package. The lines for the original stand in New York's Madison Square Park were ridiculous, and there was even a shack cam so you could go online and see exactly how long the line was.

The burger was something special. Shake Shack had enlisted wholesale meat purveyor Pat LaFrieda to create a proprietary blend of beef for Shake Shack. All of a sudden, everyone had to have a proprietary blend burger on their menu if they were going to be serious about being in the burger business.

The beef was seasoned, then smashed on a stainless-steel flat-top, cooked, and topped with cheese, lettuce, tomatoes, and ShackSauce on a buttered and toasted Martin's Potato Roll. Then it was served in a little wax bag that made it easy to eat the ShackBurger.

All I would hear about from my friends visiting New York was how the line at Shake Shack was worth the wait. I finally ate a ShackBurger at the South Beach Burger Bash in February 2010. I wasn't impressed, but a few months later when they opened up in Miami Beach, I became addicted. My wife didn't "get" the Shake Shack love I had. Then one day, all of a sudden, she was in love too.

You could tell Shake Shack was onto something as a bunch of haters started to come out of the woodwork on social media to trash them. Much like White Castle and McDonald's before them, a wave of imitators sprang up, copying details down to the color scheme, the look of the burgers, and the items on the menu.

Shake Shack has now become the gold standard. When they open up in a neighborhood, they embrace it by partnering with local businesses on dishes and using locally made products to make a special frozen custard flavor. The cult following that they initially had has gone global and is often compared to the passionate following of In-N-Out.

Shake Shack has shown us what a burger company can be, and in turn, they've kicked up the burger game to the next level. A large part of the reason for their success is the three-headed monster that is Danny Meyer (Chairman of the Board), Randy Garutti (CEO), and Mark Rosati (Culinary Director of Shake Shack), arguably the best trio in the food industry.

PS: I do not own any stock in Shake Shack.

Chapter

10

REGIONAL SPECIALTY BURGERS

Just knowing the burger joints that helped shape the history is a small part of the journey. There is much to learn and try when it comes to the diversity in styles of America's favorite sandwich.

We're going to focus on local specialty burgers. Folks in different parts of the country have made the burger their own, sometimes by just adding a topping that's popular in their neighborhoods.

California Burger

The California burger is typically topped with either avocado or its offspring, guacamole, and sometimes bacon. It's not to be confused with In-N-Out, even though that chain is synonymous with California burger culture, or what they mean when they say "California Burger" in some parts of Mississippi, where it means you want lettuce, tomato, and onion on it.

The California burger isn't too difficult to track down. I've seen the LA Burger with guac on the Bobby's Burger Palace menu and a guacamole and bacon burger on Denny's expanded menu.

Colombian "Comida Rapida" Burger

One of the advantages of living in South Florida is comfort food from Central and South America. What was street food in Colombia has found a new life in Miami in the popular quick service and late-night restaurants of Miami. It's known as "Comida Rapida," fast food.

If you like to pile on sauces, then you will find heaven on earth in the Colombian style burger. The usual suspects of lettuce, tomato, and onion top the burger, but then it's smothered in melted mozzarella cheese, crushed potato chips, and a variety of sauces.

The three most popular sauces are a creamy garlic mayo, a pink sauce which is a mix of ketchup and mayo, and a pineapple sauce. I was ready to walk out the door when they mentioned pineapple sauce, but I was wrong. It works in an indescribable way that you won't understand until you eat one of these beauties. It can be a little overwhelming on the first try, but stick with it as it gets good and addictive.

My introduction to the Colombian Burger was a tiny late-night spot named MAO which is not too far from my parent's home. My go-to for Comida Rapida is the Monster Burgers Food Truck, or on the brick-and-mortar side, Los Verdes, which has seven locations in South Florida and one in New York City.

Connecticut Steamed Cheeseburger

A stainless-steel cabinet holds mini trays for the hamburger patty and the extra melty cheddar cheese. The giant box cooks the burgers and cheese via steam generated from the basin full of water at the bottom, which is heated. Steaming gives the burgers a very meaty flavor along with a texture similar to a loose meatloaf. The patty is transferred onto a bun, then the gooey cheese is poured out on top.

Jack's Lunch from Middleton, Connecticut, is widely credited as the creator of the Steamed Cheeseburger in the late 1920s to early 1930s. Nowadays, Ted's in Meriden, Connecticut, is considered by many to be the go-to spot to grab one. Latin House in Kendall, Florida, serves them up only on Friday nights.

Dominican Chimi Burger

Santo Domingo's street food Chimi is a well-seasoned beef patty customarily shaped to the *pan de agua* (water roll) that houses it. The

Dominican pan de agua is similar to a French baguette in texture. The burger comes topped with tomato, cabbage, and salsa golf (golf sauce). While there is no clear explanation of how it ended up being called a Chimi (a shortened version of the favorite Argentinian sauce), there is a connection to that country.

Salsa golf, the original ketchup and mayo-based sauce that's all over fast food in Latin American countries, was the creation of Luis Federico Leloir of Argentina, the 1970 Nobel Prize winner for chemistry. As the story goes, he created the sauce to accompany the prawns he was enjoying at a golf club back in 1925. The original version was equal parts mayonnaise and ketchup with drops of cognac and Tabasco sauce.

I first enjoyed a Chimi years ago in a dusty lot where the Chimi Churri Los Primos food trailer sets up for late-night eats. While I don't come across Chimis on restaurant menus often, it can readily be found on many food trucks in Miami, like Chimi El Tigre and Don Mofongo.

Georgia Luther Burger

The Luther Burger is a bacon cheeseburger on glazed donuts instead of the burger buns. There's a rumor that this was created by singer Luther Vandross when he was making a cheeseburger and didn't have any type of bread at his home.

He was so starved that he chose the next best option available to him: donuts. While a great story, there's no proof that anyone ever asked him about how legit that yarn was before he died.

There is a "FatKreme" burger pictured online in 2003 with Krispy Kreme Donuts as replacement buns. It's the earliest documented proof of this burger creation that I found. While that may be true, the now closed

Mulligan's out of Decatur, Georgia, seems to have been behind the creation of the name when they added the Luther Burger to their menu in 2006.

Iowa Loose Meat Sandwiches

When David Heglin opened Ye Old Tavern in Sioux City, Iowa, in 1924, tavern burgers were on the menu. Hardcore loose meat sandwich eaters insist on calling it a Tavern or Tavern Sandwich.

These "burgers" were seasoned ground beef served up on wax paper. Two years later, Fred Angell opened up Maid-Rite and named the same dish a Maid-Rite.

Nowadays, they're mostly referred to as loose meat sandwiches and come with onions, mustard, and pickles. They are found all over Iowa, parts of Ohio and Kansas and in Detroit, Michigan, as a loose hamburger.

Michigan Olive Burger

In the 1920s, Sam Blair and his Kewpee Hotel Hamburgs numbered in the hundreds of locations. One of the more popular burgers on the menu was garnished with olives. It is not known if this was the very first Olive Burger, but Kewpee did popularize it.

You can still find this version of the sandwich at Halo Burger, the direct descendant of Blair's Kewpee restaurant locations. There are variations with an olive-based mayo spread replacing the usual spread or used in conjunction with the olives as a topping.

They are such a thing in Michigan that in 1991 Burger King tested Olive Burgers in Michigan, Ohio, and Indiana.

Minnesota Juicy Lucy

Juicy Lucy is a burger patty stuffed with a melty cheese; most of the time, it's American cheese. You need to be extra careful when taking that first bite as that molten hot magma cheese oozes out.

As the story goes, a customer at Matt's Bar & Grill asked for two hamburgers with some cheese in the middle. After biting into this new creation, he said, "That's one Juicy Lucy." The "i" was inadvertently left off the name on their menu.

Most Juicy Lucy purists feel that you need enjoy them in Minnesota. So, whether you're having a "Jucy Lucy" at Matt's Bar & Grill or a "Juicy Lucy" at the 5–8 Club, both in Minneapolis, Minnesota, OR having the "Juicy Nookie Burger" at The Nook in St. Paul, Minnesota, you'll be spiritually fulfilled.

Juicy Lucys are now found all over the US.

Mississippi Slugburger or Dough Burger

First of all, there are no slugs in a Slugburger. The name comes from the slang term for a nickel, the cost of a burger in its heyday. With that horrible thought out of the way, we can discuss it without prejudice.

Slugburgers or Dough Burgers use extenders mixed in with the meat, like bread crumbs, flour, or eggs. During World War I, and later during the Great Depression, meat was either rationed or just too expensive to buy. These fillers allowed them able to stretch the amount of beef they had.

I'm partial to the ones at Bill's Hamburgers in Amory, Mississippi, which serves theirs with mustard and onion (cheese only by request), and Phillips Grocery in Holly Springs, Mississippi, where mustard, onion, and pickle are the standard.

If you can't get enough of these, a Slugburger Festival is held yearly in Corinth, Mississippi, which also includes a Miss Slugburger pageant.

Missouri Guber Burger

The Guber Burger or Goober Burger (choose whichever spelling suits your fancy) was popularized in central Missouri by the Wheel Inn Drive-In. The local burger that I hear the most groans about is the Guber Burger, since it has a minimal appeal to the majority of the public. The Guber Burger is a burger topped with peanut butter.

The Wheel Inn Drive-In's version involved ladling or spooning warm peanut butter sauce that is almost soup-like in consistency. Unfortunately, they went out of business, and no other Guber Burger-centric restaurant has taken its place.

There are restaurants across the US that add a smear of peanut burger for a similar effect or others that serve variations on the theme, like My Sister's Place in Grand Marais, Minnesota. They kick it up a notch by topping the peanut butter with some mayo. Their version is featured on the Travel Channel's *Bizarre Foods with Andrew Zimmern*.

Montana Nutburger

I'm not the biggest fan of salted peanuts, so the thought of salted peanuts mixed with Miracle Whip topping a burger is horrifying. Some folks will try to sell you on the whole sweet and salty or crunchy and soft angle of it, but I'm not buying.

Regardless of my thoughts, people love it. You can find this unusual grub at Matt's Place Drive-In in Butte, Montana.

New Jersey-Style Slider

The origins of the New Jersey-style slider go back to a burger cooking method pioneered by White Castle's Walt Anderson. You take a ball of beef, smash it on the flat-top grill with a spatula, and top it with onions, which cook via the steam rising through the meat.

White Manna in Hackensack, New Jersey, cooks up 1½-ounce burgers in this way. When you ask for a double, you don't get two individual stacked patties. That's because they smash two balls instead of one to make a three-ouncer.

If you visit the White Rose Diner in Linden, New Jersey, they serve a larger three-ounce slider. They are also the originators of the Jersey Burger, which adds Taylor Ham, a bologna-esque sliced pork product popular with the people of New Jersey.

New Mexico Green Chile Cheeseburger

The Green Chile Cheeseburger is just that, a cheeseburger topped with chopped green chiles or a green chile sauce.

The most famous story involving the Green Chile Burger takes place in 1945 at the Owl Bar & Cafe in San Antonio, New Mexico, where the scientists from the Manhattan Project were rumored to be enjoying them nightly after long days working on the atomic bomb.

Its popularity has spawned a New Mexico Green Chile Cheese Trail online where you can make your way around the state from one spot to another sampling this specialty at various burger joints. And yes, the Owl Bar & Cafe is still around.

Oklahoma City Theta Burger

At some point between the 1930s and 1940, the Theta Burger was born when a place called Town Tavern created a signature burger for the Kappa Alpha Theta sorority at the University of Oklahoma. The burger features a hickory BBQ sauce, pickles, mayonnaise, and shredded cheddar cheese.

When the Town Tavern closed, the scoreboards with the OU football game information were moved to The Mont near the university. Of course, you can find a Theta Burger at The Mont and at Johnnie's Charcoal Broiler locations near Oklahoma City, Oklahoma.

Oklahoma Fried Onion Burger

If you're into grilled onions, then the Oklahoma Fried Onion Burger has your name all over it. During the Depression, ground beef was expensive. At this time, burgers had just turned the corner after their revived popularity, sparked partially by White Castle.

According to John T. Edge, Ross Davis would smash onions into his burgers to give his customers more bang for their buck with a bigger patty. His restaurant, the Hamburger Inn, was located at the intersection of Route 66 and Highway 81 in Oklahoma. Due to its central proximity, other establishments in the El Reno area began serving the fried onion burger. I know many folks who swear by this burger, and that includes my burger mentor George Motz. George makes a pretty mean version of the fried onion burger.

Patty Melt

A Patty Melt is the perfect example of a burger sandwich. A topic that comes up often is whether or not a Patty Melt should be classified as a burger. I've always felt that a Patty Melt was a burger, not so much a sandwich, if that makes any sense.

The "official" ingredients are simple: Burger patty, rye bread, Swiss cheese, and grilled onions.

I can't say that I ever remember eating a bad one anywhere, and I've had my fill of them in many cities and states. Assuming all the proper items are in place., it's almost impossible to mess one up.

I do encounter variations on the cheeses (American or cheddar), or occasionally on the bread (sourdough or Texas toast), but rarely on the protein, although I've had a "Turkey" Patty Melt.

Most Patty Melt purists say that the rye bread is never to be toasted, only griddled on the flat-top. The Patty Melt should taste like the child of a great burger and a grilled cheese sandwich.

You can now find Patty Melts on menus across the US, but it was initially a California creation. It is believed that the papa was Tiny Naylor, who owned a chain of Biff's and Tiny Naylor restaurants in the late 1940s and 1950s in California.

Tiny passed in 1959, but his son Biff (yes, the restaurants were named after him) now owns the Du-Par's chain, which has a great Patty Melt on the menu. His granddaughter Jennifer, now a caterer, was formerly an executive chef for Wolfgang Puck.

Pimento Cheese Burger

Pimento Cheese, the beautiful marriage of shredded cheese, mayo, and diced pimento peppers, is a favorite topping on many foods in the South and, most importantly, on burgers.

Finding a restaurant that serves a Pimento Cheese Burger can be as easy as just finding one that has pimento cheese on the menu. Burgers will follow shortly after.

You're more likely to encounter them when driving around the South in the US. I still fantasize about the fantastic Pimento Cheese Burger from Boyce General Store in Alvaton, Kentucky.

San Antonio Bean Burger

The San Antonio Bean Burger makes its home mostly in and around San Antonio, Texas. The best-known version of it is a burger patty topped with refried beans, Cheez Whiz, crushed Fritos, and diced onions.

Different interpretations of the Bean Burger now exist, like the Tostada Burger at Chris Madrid's, where the Cheez Whiz is replaced by cheddar cheese and the Fritos by homemade chips.

Tennessee Deep Fried Burger

When it comes to deep fried burgers, Dyer's in Memphis, Tennessee, is the first spot that comes to mind for most people. Dyer's claim to fame? They've never thrown out the grease they use to fry the burgers. The "Vitamin G," as it is known, is strained daily.

What they do at Dyer's is smash down a patty until it's wafer-thin, then drop it ever so gently into the prehistoric oil. It will sink and then float to the top to signify that it's good to go. Initially, I was confident that I would be having the greasiest meat patty known to man, but I was wrong. If you need more of that Vitamin G, you can ask to have it dunked, bread and all.

Just over the Tennessee border in Tompkinsville, Kentucky, you will find Dovie's. They submerge their burgers in soybean oil, giving it a nice crispy exterior. Just drop the term "squozed" to them, and they drain your patty of all the excess fat.

Utah Pastrami Burger

Whoever thought of topping their cheeseburger with pastrami deserves a monument. There is no official creator, but in Salt Lake City, Utah, with their Greek diners and restaurants, burgers covered with pastrami, thousand island dressing, and cheese do not sound out of the ordinary.

Crown Burgers was flying the flag for pastrami burgers in 1978 when they opened in Salt Lake City. Back then, only a few sold each day, but now it's their top-selling item.

Wisconsin Butter Burger

The first time I laid eyes on a Butter Burger, I was innocently watching George Motz's documentary *Hamburger America*; in it, he profiled Solly's Grille in Milwaukee, Wisconsin.

I had never seen anything like it before. Just like all great burger spots, they use a fresh, never frozen beef patty. After doing the customary sandwich setup, they finish it up with a massive smear of butter and then the top bun. The butter melts and cascades down all the sides of this now majestic dish. I might be overselling it, but I rewound and watched it a few times to take in what I was seeing.

The Butter Burger is mostly found in and around Wisconsin, although the Culver's chain has been spreading the name statewide.

How to make a Butter Burger varies. There's the method used by Solly's Grille (who created it in 1936); just having the butter as a topping on the burger, or the butter can be added to the burger patty itself.

The one tip I can leave you with when you encounter a Butter Burger is to eat it fast, or you're going to have a giant mess on your hands. I'm also pretty sure it's in the burger eating handbook that all butter pooling at the bottom of your plate automatically becomes a burger dipping sauce.

Wisconsin Poached Burger

Another unique burger in the US is the Poached Burger found at Pete's Hamburgers. They've served this delicacy since 1909 in Prairie du Chien, Wisconsin. Pete's is only open Fridays, Saturdays, and Sundays from May to October. The exact day of the month they open varies by the year based on the weather.

The Poached Burger starts with a four-ounce ball of beef that is smashed onto the flat-top grill, then cooked in boiling water filled with onions. The end product is a very juicy patty. Your only options when it comes to toppings is with or without onions, with no cheese whatsoever.

Chapter
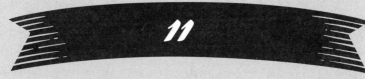
11

LA FRITA CUBANA

The Frita or Frita Cubana is originally from Cuba but predominantly found in Miami. It is a regional burger and was originally going to be part of that chapter. But when I was writing this book, I uncovered enough new information to expand it. Below you will find the history of a burger that I hold near and dear to my heart, La Frita Cubana.

FRITA CUBANA HISTORY

The earliest known mention of the word *frita* was in 1923 in the Cuban slang dictionary N*uevo Catauro de Cubanismos* by the author Fernando Ortiz. The Frita is described as a type of sandwich with ground beef, onion, and fried potatoes between two pieces of bread. A key ingredient not mentioned in the definition is smoked paprika (*pimentón*), which gives the Frita that distinct taste.

The Frita was sold in Cuba by "*Friteros*" from their sidewalk stands, which were called "*Puestos.*" They were cooked over small portable stoves. Today's hot dog stands are a reasonable basis for comparison. Their popularity was attributed to its mobile nature. Most kids would get out of school and go by the Fritero to eat a Frita on the way home. Adults also got into the action by stopping for a snack on the way to a movie theater. The Frita is remembered by most folks as an essential part of their interaction with the community in Cuba.

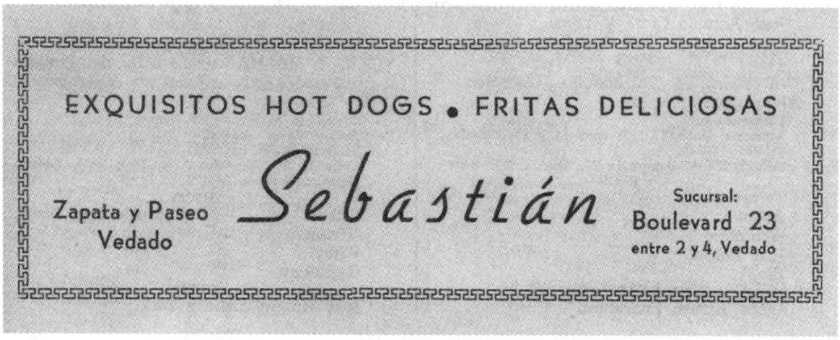

197

EXQUISITOS HOT DOGS • FRITAS DELICIOSAS

Zapata y Paseo
Vedado

Sebastián

Sucursal:
Boulevard 23
entre 2 y 4, Vedado

Only known advertisement for a Frita stand in Cuba from the
Libro de Oro de la Sociedad Habanera 1958.

In 1961, Ramon Estevill and his sons Dagoberto, Tomas, Daniel, and Miguel decided to sell Fritas in the Little Havana part of Miami via a cart similar to the ones that lined Havana, Cuba. While living in Cuba, Dagoberto had been a car salesman at his father's business, but he had befriended Bebo, the son of Havana's most famous Fritero (Frita maker), Sebastián Carro Seijido. He learned everything about how to make a Frita from scratch from him, including the preparation of the julienne potatoes that are the real secret to mastering a great Frita recipe.

By March, 1962, they had opened the fourteen-seat brick-and-mortar Fritas Domino in the Little Havana part of Miami. It brought much emotional comfort to those fleeing from Cuba to Miami for what they thought would be a temporary thing. Fritas Domino went on to open three more locations over the next three years with the fourth and final one opening in Hialeah, Florida, in 1965. I also loved their catchphrase, "¡Si te come una, te come dos!" which means if you eat one, you've gotta eat two of them.

In late 1962, the Morro Castle corporation was incorporated, but it was not until January of 1963 that Morro Castle opened its doors in a former

Dairy Isle building. Alberto Villalobos and his partner added some tables around the open-air counter and converted it into a drive-in.

The Morro Castle menu from 1964 featured a fifteen-cent Frita Cubana, a twenty-five cent Perro Caliente (hot dog), a fifteen-cent "Hamburguer" and twenty-cent cheeseburgers. This same year Alberto, now the sole owner, bought the property.

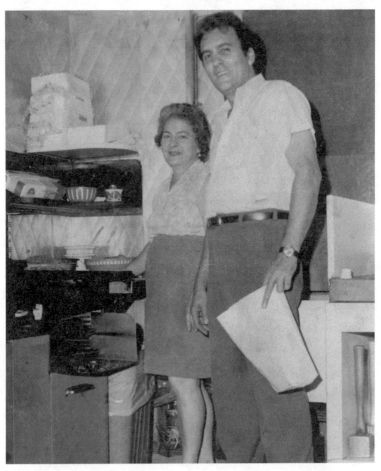

Morro Castle founder Alberto Villalobos with employee in the kitchen circa late 1960s.

The second Morro Castle location was built in east Hialeah and opened in late 1966. Alberto split his time running both places until his brother Horacio Villalobos arrived from Cuba with his family in early 1967. The original location on NW 7th Street would prepare the uncooked Frita patties, churros, and flans for both restaurants. It operated as a commissary for both locations until 1984, when Alberto passed away.

On March 13, 1968, all privately owned businesses were shut down in Cuba as part of a "Revolutionary Offensive," and that, of course, included Frita stands, leaving Miami as the only place to find the former street food.

The Cuban exile community continued to enjoy Fritas at cafeterias, predominantly patronized by those who had settled in the part of Miami that would come to be called Little Havana. This was a hotbed for Frita activity, including spots like Rolando Botana's El Coladito. He once disclosed that his secret Frita recipe included ground beef, ground pork, vinegar, garlic, paprika, and a few other spices.

Other contemporaries included Badias, El Palacio de las Fritas (Palace of the Fritas), and El Rey de las Fritas (King of the Fritas); they were all known for their Fritas, but only El Rey de las Fritas has stood the test of time.

Ramon Estevill passed away in 1980, and a few years later his sons decided to sell the business, but not the name and brand. The location at 1177 SW 8th Street would eventually fall into the hands of Victoriano "Benito" Gonzalez, who had sold Fritas in Placetas, Cuba, until 1968. Benito was already part of the El Palacio de las Fritas restaurant with some partners at this point.

He asked his brother-in-law Ortelio Cardenas and his sister Eva to move from New Jersey to help him run this new spot. Ortelio, who had never worked in the food business, decided to make a career change. They relocated with their children Frank and Martha to Miami. Benito taught Ortelio everything he knew about the food industry and how to run a restaurant.

El Rey de las Fritas opened in the former Fritas Domino space and popularized the Frita to those outside the Cuban community. During this time, Ortelio added cheese to the Frita in an attempt to "Americanize" it. (Just an FYI: Fritas with cheese are frowned upon by hardcore and old-school Frita fans.)

Once Benito finished up his other Frita responsibilities, he and Ortelio were under the same roof. It wasn't long before Ortelio and his wife Eva made their own way. On September 12, 1984, El Mago de las Fritas opened in West Miami. *El Mago*, or the magician, as Ortelio was called, took everything he learned from the Frita King and put his own twist on things.

Benito passed away in 2005 and leave El Rey de las Fritas in the more than capable hands of his wife Angelina, son Yamil, and daughter Mercedes. Angelina runs the *Calle Ocho* location, while Mercedes and her husband Gino are at the El Rey de las Fritas locations in Hialeah and Sweetwater. Yamil's El Rey de las Fritas restaurant can be found on a busy strip mall corner in the Westchester part of Miami where I grew up.

Morro Castle in Hialeah relocated after Alberto's passing on September 14, 1984. It would now operate independently from the original location in Little Havana run by Horacio and Leonardo Villalobos. Alberto senior's wife and his son Alberto soldiered on at the first spot until Alberto the son and his wife (Alberto senior's daughter-in-law) took over.

A Miami Herald article from 1987 mentioned that the first Morro Castle went through seven hundred pounds of julienne potatoes, six hundred pounds of bread, and ten thousand Fritas on average weekly. That's just insane.

In 1987, Fritas Domino, then run by Dagoberto Estevill, reopened in West Miami near the former site of a Palacio de las Fritas and right down the street from El Mago de las Fritas.

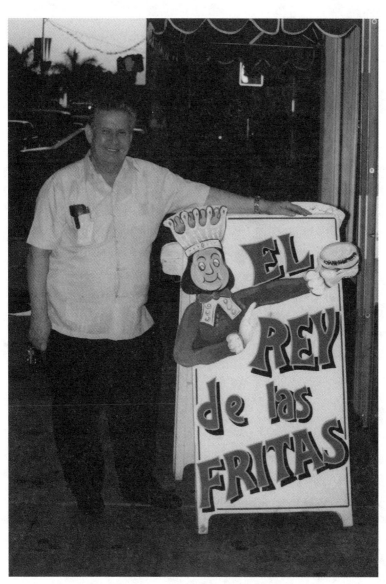

Victoriano "Benito" Gonzalez, founder of El Rey de las Fritas, standing next to a sign he painted in the late 1990s.

Two events finally caused the Frita to break through to a broader audience. The first occurred in October, 2010, when President Obama stopped in at El Mago and grabbed one Frita and five Fritas with cheese to go while he famously drank the Cuban soft drink Materva on his way out. I was there right after Secret Service allowed folks back into the neighborhood, and El Mago was swarmed with customers. The next day, I hung out most of the day there, and the bread delivery was hours late. He was down to less than a dozen Cuban rolls, and I went to find some and returned with three garbage bags full of rolls. I had taken so much bread from a bakery down the street, they had no means to package it, which is why they ended up in garbage bags. It was utter madness.

What really made the Frita start to spread nationwide and worldwide was the appearance of El Mago de las Fritas and El Rey de las Fritas on the Travel Channel program *Burger Land*, hosted by George Motz. George did a great job explaining the history of the Frita and featuring the two restaurant's histories. The episode is out there, so track it down, 'cause you'll catch me with George having Fritas at El Mago.

After more than fifty years, Little Havana's Morro Castle closed on June 15, 2017, in a blow to the soul of the Frita community. Luckily, there is a very strong rumor that Alberto is looking to reopen and bring it back.

Over the last couple of years, second and third generation Cubans who grew up in Miami have started to serve up their take on the Frita Cubana. You can find excellent Fritas which are not quite old-school but do have a little bit of that magic in them at places like Amelia's 1931, Ariete, Cao Bakery & Cafe, and Off the Mile in Miami, or the A Lo Cubano Kitchen Food Truck in Orlando, Florida. While you're at it, I suggest you track down my friend Barry Hennessey (better known as El Gringo de las Fritas) who is always trying something new with the Frita.

When you visit my hometown of Miami, Florida, make sure to visit Fritas Domino, Morro Castle, Sergio's, El Rey de las Fritas, El Mago de las Fritas, and Cuban Guys (listed in order of when they were established, not alphabetically) for a real deal Frita experience.

If you're ever in the neighborhood, on Saturday mornings you're likely to catch me hanging with Ortelio and his daughter Martha at El Mago de las Fritas for breakfast.

I know it's not possible for everyone to have an authentic Frita experience, which is why I've included my recipe so that you can make one at home.

Burger Beast's Frita Cubana Recipe

Serves five.

INGREDIENTS

- 1 pound of 80/20 chuck
- 3 tablespoons smoked Spanish paprika
- 2 teaspoons granulated garlic powder
- 1 teaspoon onion powder
- ¼ teaspoon cumin
- 1 tablespoon Crystal hot sauce
- 1 large yellow onion, diced
- 1 cup of cooking oil, or as needed
- 2 medium russet potatoes
- Ideally 5 Cuban bread rolls, but French bread rolls or regular soft, squishy hamburger rolls will do

DIRECTIONS

1. Shred the two potatoes on a cheese grater, then rinse them thoroughly until the water is clear.

2. Drain and squeeze dry on paper towels. To get them really crispy, you need to remove as much moisture as possible.

3. Add the cooking oil to a non-stick pan and heat to medium high. Add the potatoes and let them cook until they are crispy.

4. Let the potatoes dry on paper towels and season with salt according to your taste.

   Getting the julienne potatoes right is the most difficult part of the recipe, but there's a little cheat. Go to your local grocer and purchase Ore-Ida "Shredded Hash Brown Potatoes" instead.

DIRECTIONS

5. Mix the smoked Spanish paprika, garlic powder, onion powder, cumin, and Crystal hot sauce into the ground chuck.

6. Make five equally sized balls of the seasoned meat.

7. Take one of the Frita-seasoned balls of beef, and using a thick spatula, smash onto a cast-iron skillet on a burner at medium high heat.

8. Grab a respectable large pinch of diced onions and place on the smashed patty.

9. Add salt as you would to any burger that you're cooking.

10. After cooking for approximately forty-five seconds to a minute, flip the Frita onto the onion side to finish.

11. Place the bottom bun on the Frita while it's finishing and let it warm a little bit.*

12. Slide the spatula under the deliciousness and flip it so that the bottom bun is resting on your hand with the Frita and onions on top.

13. At this point, you can choose to add some raw diced onions and maybe a little dash of ketchup to bring out the flavor of the patty and the julienne potatoes.

14. All that's left to do is add the top bun, and you're good to go!

* You can toast the buns lightly beforehand if you have the time or as a matter of preference.

Chapter

12

BURGER COMPETITIONS

There are so many burger-related events that you could keep yourself busy year-round attending them. Some are competitions to find the best in a region; a few celebrate historical burger events or regional burger specialties; but the one important thing they have in common is that they celebrate the burger.

Here are some of the must-attend bashes, battles, festivals, and parties.

Burger Fest

Homeofthehamburger.org

The Burger Fest of Seymour, Wisconsin, just celebrated its thirtieth year in August 2018. "Hamburger Charlie" Nagreen's claim to the invention of the hamburger is the driving force behind this fest. Some of the things that you can expect are a Burger Fest car show, a giant ketchup slide, a burger eating contest, and the cooking of the two hundred-pound giant hamburger. It all gets started with the world's largest hamburger parade.

BurgerFest

Hamburgburgerfest.com

The first BurgerFest coincided with the hundred-year anniversary of the Menches' claim to the naming of the hamburger in 1985. The Hamburg Chamber of Commerce, which created the event, read about the Menches and thought it would make a great community happening. The one-day event features music, entertainment, and of course, burgers. BurgerFest is generally held on the third Saturday of July in Hamburg, New York.

Cheeseburger in Caseville

Casevillechamber.com

The inaugural Caseville Cheeseburger Festival was a three-day event in Caseville, Michigan, created by local Lyn Bezemek in 1999. Cheeseburger is in the title, but there's a little more depth to this event, as it also glorifies the Jimmy Buffet laid-back "Cheeseburger in Paradise" lifestyle. The cheeseburger eating contest and the "Best Cheeseburger" award for local businesses fulfill its burger event requirements, while the Parade of Tropical Fools adds some fun. The Caseville Cheeseburger Festival is now a ten-day party in mid to late August that draws well over one hundred thousand attendees.

Denver Burger Battle

Denverburgerbattle.com

The Denver Burger Battle happens every August in Denver, Colorado. Founded by Jeremy Kossler, it features approximately fifteen different local burger restaurants competing for the People's Choice and Judge's Choice awards.

2018 People's Choice: Hearth & Dram
2018 Judge's Choice: Stanley Beer Hall

2017 People's Choice: Stoic & Genuine
2017 Judge's Choice: Stanley Beer Hall

2016 People's Choice: Cherry Cricket
2016 Judge's Choice: Stoic & Genuine

2015 People's Choice: TAG Burger Bar
2015 Judge's Choice: The Nickel

2014 People's Choice: Crave Real Burgers

2014 Judge's Choice: Crave Real Burgers

2013 People's Choice: TAG Burger Bar

2013 Judge's Choice: Park Burger

2012 People's Choice: Crave Real Burgers

2012 Judge's Choice: Larkburger

2011 People's Choice: Highland Tap and Burger

2011 Judge's Choice: Park Burger

2010 People's Choice: H Burger

2010 Judge's Choice: Park Burger

El Reno Burger Day Festival

Elrenoburgerday.com

The El Reno Burger Day Festival was created to cook the world's largest fried onion hamburger. The first fest in May 1989 featured Sid's Diner, Johnnie's Grill, and Robert's Grill selling their fried onion burgers. The sheer number of people who showed up to support their local fried onion hamburger joints was overwhelming, and now, almost thirty years later, it draws over twenty-five thousand attendees. "Burger Day" is celebrated every May in El Reno, Oklahoma, and still features the cooking of the world's largest fried onion hamburger. In 2018, it weighed in at 850 lbs.

Frita Showdown

Fritashowdown.com

Frita Showdown is one of a handful of burger competitions that revolves around a regional specialty, the Frita Cubana. I've been writing about and singing the praises of this Cuban street food staple since the very beginning of my food blog more than ten years ago. I created the Frita Showdown in 2013 to give the Frita Cubana a well-deserved day in the spotlight.

At the first event, I dedicated the Frita Showdown to the memory of my maternal grandparents, Gregorio and Juana Echevarria, who left behind oppression in Cuba looking for a better life for my family. Nothing has changed, except it's now dedicated to anyone who sacrificed themselves for their family by coming to the United States, even if it meant starting all over.

Hamburger House Party

Hamburgerhouseparty.com

Hamburger House Party was initially known as the Burger Beast Burger Brawl but underwent a name change after its second year. The event's founder is Sef "Burger Beast" Gonzalez, a.k.a. me, and we hold the event in Miami, Florida, during the spring. The number of competitors going after the People's and Judge's Choice awards is right around twenty restaurants. Each year we feature locals as well as a few out-of-towners.

2018 People's Choice: Hate Mondays Tavern

2018 Judge's Choice: Jr's Gourmet Burgers

2017 People's Choice: Chefs on the Run

2017 Judge's Choice: Hard Times Sundaes (Brooklyn, New York)

2016 People's Choice: Jr's Gourmet Burgers

2016 Judge's Choice: Burbowl

2015 People's Choice: Jr's Gourmet Burgers

2014 People's Choice: Latin House

National Hamburger Festival

Hamburgerfestival.com

Much like BurgerFest, the National Hamburger Festival was inspired by the Menches' claim to the invention of the hamburger. Drew Cerza founded the event in Akron, Ohio, where it still makes its home every summer. Over twenty thousand festivalgoers attend the two-day event, which features twenty restaurants serving different styles of hamburgers, a Miss Hamburger pageant, the Ohio Hamburger Eating Championship, and a hamburger cook-off.

New York City Wine & Food Festival Burger Bash

Nycwff.org/burger

The New York City Wine & Food Festival Burger Bash happens every October in New York. The founders of the NYCWFF Burger Bash are Lee Brian Schrager and Rachael Ray, and it is produced by Randy Fisher and his company CREaM (Culinary Related Entertainment and Marketing). It features restaurants from the New York area and beyond, with some food celebrity names thrown into the mix. The sister event to this competition happens in South Beach.

2018 People's Choice: Clinton Hall
2018 Judge's Choice: Citi Field

2017 People's Choice: Black Tap Craft Burgers & Beer
2017 Judge's Choice: Le Rivage

2016 People's Choice: Black Tap Craft Burgers & Beer
2016 Judge's Choice: David's Café

2015 People's Choice: Black Tap Craft Burgers & Beer

2015 Judge's Choice: BBD's Beers, Burgers, Desserts

2014 People's Choice: Burger & Barrel

2014 Judge's Choice: Landmarc

2013 People's Choice TIE: Burger & Barrel and Guy Fieri

2013 Judge's Choice: Le Rivage

2012 People's Choice: Burger & Barrel

2012 Judge's Choice: Ai Fiori

2011 People's Choice: Burger & Barrel

2011 Judge's Choice: Abe & Arthurs

2010 People's Choice: Bobby's Burger Palace (Paramus, New Jersey)

2010 Judge's Choice: Shake Shack

2009 People's Choice: Lure

2009 Judge's Choice: Good Stuff Eatery (Washington, DC)

2008 People's Choice: Katie Lee Joel

Sacramento Burger Battle

Sacburgerbattle.com

My burger brother Rodney Blackwell founded the Sacramento Burger Battle. It features fifteen of the best burger restaurants in the Sacramento, California, area competing for People's Choice and Judge's Choice awards. Rodney's oldest daughter was diagnosed with Crohn's disease, so all funds raised from the event benefit the Crohn's & Colitis Foundation.

2018 People's Choice: Pangaea Cafe

2018 Judge's Choice: Pangaea Cafe

2017 People's Choice: Dawson's Steakhouse

2017 Judge's Choice: Empress Tavern

2016 People's Choice: LowBrau

2016 Judge's Choice: Pangaea Cafe

2015 People's Choice: Dawson's Steakhouse

2015 Judge's Choice: Pangaea Cafe

2014 People's Choice: de Vere's Irish Pub

2014 Judge's Choice: Dawson's Steakhouse

2013 People's Choice: Broderick Roadhouse

2013 Judge's Choice: Ettore's

2012 People's Choice: Krush Burger

2012 Judge's Choice: The Chef's Tables

Slugburger Festival

Slugburgerfestival.com

Every July, the Slugburger Festival celebrates you guessed it...the Slugburger, a unique regional burger. This weekend festival was founded more than thirty years ago in Corinth, Mississippi. True to its burger origins, the Slugburger Festival features a carnival. Live music, Slugburgers, and the Miss Slugburger pageant are a part of the yearly celebration. The World Slugburger Eating Contest, currently on hiatus, can lay claim to having professional eaters Joey Chestnut and Matt Stonie as previous winners.

South Beach Wine & Food Festival Burger Bash

Sobewff.org/burgerbash

The South Beach & Food Festival Burger Bash happens every February in Miami Beach, Florida. Considered by many (including me) to be the burger competition which set the standard for everyone, the South Beach Burger Bash was founded by Lee Brian Schrager and Rachael Ray, and it is produced by Randy Fisher and his company CREaM. The restaurants featured are both from South Florida and from out of state burger joints, along with some food celebrities. It predates its sister event in New York by one year.

2018 People's Choice: Swine Southern Table & Bar
2018 Judge's Choice: Butter (New York, New York)

2017 People's Choice: Jr's Gourmet Burgers
2017 Judge's Choice: Little Jack's Tavern (Charleston, South Carolina)

2016 People's Choice: Morimoto
2016 Judge's Choice: Jersey Dawg

2015 People's Choice: Pincho Factory
2015 Judge's Choice: Lure Fishbar

2014 People's Choice: B Spot (Cleveland, Ohio)
2014 Judge's Choice: Shake Shack

2013 People's Choice: Bobby's Burger Palace
2013 Judge's Choice: Jeff Mauro

2012 People's Choice: B Spot (Cleveland, Ohio)
2012 Judge's Choice: Whisk

2011 People's Choice: B Spot (Cleveland, Ohio)

2011 Judge's Choice: Landmarc (New York, New York)

2010 People's Choice: B Spot (Cleveland, Ohio)

2010 Judge's Choice: Michael's Genuine Food & Drink

2009 People's Choice: Good Stuff Eatery (Washington, DC)

2009 Judge's Choice: Good Stuff Eatery (Washington, DC)

2008 People's Choice: Radius (Boston, Massachusetts)

2007 People's Choice: Shake Shack (New York, New York)

Taste of Hamburg-er Festival

Tasteofhamburger.com

Hamburg, Pennsylvania, throws the massive Taste of Hamburg-er Festival every year. Its estimated attendance for its fifteenth anniversary in 2018 was almost fifty thousand; that's a whole lot of burger fans in one place. It has grown from three blocks to eight blocks and features an amateur and professional burger eating competition as well as over thirty burger stands and live music.

2018 Best Burger Restaurant: Spuds

2018 Best Burger Organization: Salem Church

2018 Burger Mobile Unit: Blazing Swine BBQ

2017 Best Burger Restaurant: Bull and Bear Restaurant

2017 Best Burger Organization: Christ Evangelical Free Church

2017 Burger Mobile Unit: Uncle Paul's Stuffed Pretzels

2016 Best Burger Restaurant: Dawn's Deli

2016 Best Burger Organization: Christ Evangelical Free Church

2016 Burger Mobile Unit: Smokin' Bull Shack

2015 Best Burger Restaurant: Kooper's Chowhound

2015 Best Burger Organization: Salem EC Church

2015 Burger Mobile Unit: Ray's Catering

2014 Best Burger Restaurant: Smokin' Bull Shack

2014 Best Burger Organization: Salem EC Church

Uncle Fletch Hamburger Festival

Unclefletchfestival.com

The Uncle Fletch Hamburger Festival was inspired by Fletcher Davis' 1904 claim to being the creator of the hamburger. The first one took place in Athens after the Texas Legislature proclaimed Athens, Texas, to be the "Official Home of the Hamburger." There are cook-offs for the greatest hamburgers and the best hamburger side dish, along with contests like bobbing for burgers in ketchup and live entertainment. Make sure to mark September on your calendar if this sounds like the event for you.

Last Burger Bite

All of my early burger memories are tied to members of my family. When I was growing up, my dad worked for WISE potato chips. I spent my summer vacations working with him. I ate my first Frita Cubana at Morro Castle in Hialeah on our lunch break when he wanted to introduce me to something that he had enjoyed in Cuba when he was a kid.

Every year for my birthday, we would go out to celebrate. I was so obsessed with G.A.B.E.'s Burgers and Fries in Westchester, Florida, that I convinced my family to stay home instead of going out of town. My dad and I went through their double drive-thru to pick up enough food for all of us.

By the time I hit sixth grade, I was sick of watching kids coming back from summer vacation with a Hard Rock Cafe T-shirt and telling me how great the burgers were. I knew that we were visiting my dad's mom, a.k.a. my other grandmother, in Glendale, California, the following summer. So I begged my parents to take me to the Hard Rock in Los Angeles. My wish was granted. That was the same summer that I first ate at Carl's Jr, In-N-Out, Jack in the Box, and Original Tommy's World Famous Hamburgers.

When Burger King announced that it was opening a Whopper Bar in Orlando with a make your own Whopper and beer in bottles on the menu, I knew I had to visit. I woke up early with my sister-in-law Milagros in tow and drove three and a half hours just to say I had visited.

Those are just a small part of my burger memories over the years.

I hope that you learned something new about a restaurant that you loved growing up. I hope this book brought back fond memories of visits to drive-ins for a frosty root beer with your pops or maybe enjoying a snack at the luncheonette after a day of shopping with your mom.

One last thing...I want you to close your eyes and think about your fondest memories with burgers. Now, wasn't that great?

Acknowledgments

The real truth is this book would not have been possible without the help and support of these folks.

My wife Marcela who had to deal with all of my sleepless nights and did a great job of pretending to be excited whenever I told her about a new detail I had discovered. My parents Cary and Serafin Gonzalez who at a moment's notice would drop whatever they were doing to help me out.

Gretchen Schmidt is one of the kindest people I have met since my life as Burger Beast began over ten years ago. She is also a very talented editor who helped me out immensely. "Miami" Mike Hiscano, Phillip Pessar, and "Guayaba" Jorge Zaldivar who continue to assist me with research and unearthing long forgotten food history.

I love A&W Restaurants (Liz Bazner & Pete Knight), Dog 'n Suds (David Hosticka), Druther's (Brian Easley), McDonald's (Peter J. Menendez, Pepe Montes, and Bryan Rodriguez), Wendy's (Bry Toth) and White Castle (Jamie Richardson) for taking the time to talk to me and help me out in any way they could.

La Frita Cubana chapter was a labor of love and Alberto Villalobos from Morro Castle, Barry Hennessey, Mercy Gonzalez from El Rey de las Fritas and Ortelio Cardenas "El Mago de las Fritas" helped me to dot the i's and cross the t's on the history of this beloved regional specialty. Also thanks to Mike Lugo who is responsible for all the cool graphics associated with Burger Beast including the burger on the cover of this book.

My peeps from Mango Publishing, from the marketing department to the editors, including, of course, Hugo Villabona for believing in your friendly neighborhood Burger Beast.

I can't forget all these folks: My family (Alexandra Echevarria, Freddy Soler, Efrain Sequeira, Manny Perez, and of course, my sister, Michelle

Lynn Gonzalez), the older brother I always wanted, John Colella, Magic City Casino (Scott Savin, Anthony Mateo, Yadelin Crespo, and Will Bartram), Alejandro "Nike" Rodriguez, Alfredo Hernandez, Angel Abreu, "Gerther" Edric Estevez, Jimmy Piedrahita (I gave him a wedgie and stuffed him in a locker), baby face Jochi Hernandez, my brother from another mother Mark Custin, Chef Michell Sanchez, Mad Scientist Nedal Ahmad, Steve Simon (I stuffed him in a locker too) and certainly least, I mean certainly not least the Foodie Mayor, Zavier Garcia,

One last one to the late great Don Boyd who's tireless work in keeping history alive was infectious. This one's for you Bubba!

Bibliography

Aaseng, Nathan, *Business Builders in Fast Food* (2001)

Carey, Bill, *Fortunes, Fiddles & Fried Chicken: A Nashville Business History* (2004)

Cronin, Robert P., *Selling Steakburgers: The Growth of a Corporate Culture* (2000)

Edge, John T., *Hamburgers & Fries: An American Story* (2005)

Hirschorn, Paul and Steven Izenour, *White Towers* (2007)

Hogan, David Gerard, *Selling 'em by the Sack* (1997)

Ingram, E.W. Sr., *All This from a 5-cent Hamburger!: The Story of the White Castle System* (1964)

Jakle, John A. and Keith A. Sculle, *Fast Food: Roadside Restaurants in the Automobile Age* (1999)

Kroc, Ray, *Grinding It Out: The Making of McDonald's* (1977)

Love, John F., *McDonald's: Behind the Arches* (1995)

McDonald, John P., *Flameout: The Rise and Fall of Burger Chef* (2011)

McLamore, James W., *The Burger King: Jim McLamore and the Building of an Empire* (1997)

Motz, George, *Hamburger America: A State-By-State Guide to 200 Great Burger Joints* (2016)

Ozersky, Josh, *The Hamburger* (2008)

Perman, Stacy, *In-N-Out Burger* (2009)

Rozin, Elisabeth, *The Primal Cheeseburger* (1994)

Sammarco, Anthony Mitchell, *A History of Howard Johnson's: How a Massachusetts Soda Fountain Became an American Icon* (2013)

Smith, Andrew F., *Hamburger: A Global History* (2008)

Swilik, Gary, *West Side Cleveland Restaurants* (2012)

Tennyson, Jeffrey, *Hamburger Heaven* (1993)

Thomas, R. David, *Dave's Way* (1991)

White Castle, *By the Sackful* (2005)

Illustration Credits

A&W Drive-In picture courtesy of A&W Restaurants

Bob Wian picture courtesy of the Bruce B. Hermann Collection

Burger Castle picture courtesy of Joe Wasik

Burger King picture courtesy of David R. Edgerton

Burger Queen picture courtesy of State Archives of Florida/Steinmetz

Carl's Hot Dog Stand and Hardee's pictures courtesy of CKE Restaurants

Clara Peller and Dave Thomas pictures courtesy of Wendy's

El Rey de las Fritas, Benito Gonzalez picture courtesy of the El Rey de
  las Fritas family

Krystal picture courtesy of Krystal Restaurants

Morro Castle's Alberto Villalobos picture courtesy of the Villalobos family

White Castle picture courtesy of White Castle and the Ohio History Collection

Carrol's Grand Opening Ad, Fritero Sebastián Ad, Hamburger Stand
  Postcard, Kewpee Hotel Hamburg picture, McDonald's Fries Ad, Royal
  Castle Grand Opening Ad, White Tower, and Woolworth pictures are
  part of the ephemera on display at Burger Beast's Burger Museum in
  Miami, Florida.

About the Author

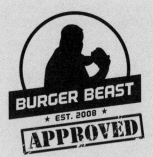

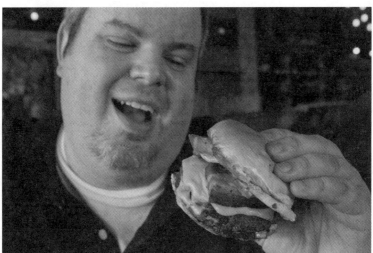

Sef Gonzalez, better known as Burger Beast, started his blog in September of 2008 with the hope of documenting his burger excursions around South Florida and beyond. The Beast began to branch out beyond burgers and cover all facets of comfort food, along with some food history mixed in whenever and wherever his journeys took him.

He then turned his eyes toward culinary events, including the first food truck event in the State of Florida. The Beast and his wife Marcela curate and produce social food gatherings throughout the year, like Frita Showdown and Hamburger House Party.

After a vintage Burger Chef sign was gifted to him, it awakened a long dormant need to find out more about the history of restaurants. Over the course of eight years he has amassed a collection of artifacts and ephemera extending from restaurants' golden age to the present. The Beast's collection now numbers over five thousand pieces and is on display at his Burger Museum in Miami, Florida.

You can continue to follow his exploits as **@BurgerBeast** on social media and on his blog: **https://burgerbeast.com/**